Full-Frontal Edition
The Naked Truth About PERIMENOPAUSE

Full-Frontal Edition

The Naked Truth About PERIMENOPAUSE

SUSANNE MITCHELL

What women (and those who love them)
need to know about the transition to menopause

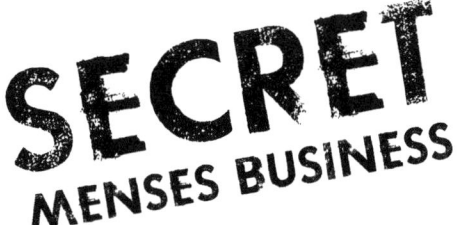

www.nakedtruthbooks.com

#secretmensesbusiness #rockingmymidlife #wisewomenrising

The Naked Truth About PERIMENOPAUSE

First published 2021 by Naked Truth Books
PO Box 640
Terrey Hills NSW 2084
Australia
www.nakedtruthbooks.com

© Susanne Mitchell 2020
www.susanne-mitchell.com

The moral right of Susanne Mitchell to be identified as the author of this work has been asserted. All rights reserved. Apart from any fair dealing for the purpose of private study, research, criticism or review, as permitted under the Copyright Act, no part of this book may be reproduced, stored in or introduced into a retrieval system, or transmitted in any form, or by any means (electronic, mechanical, photocopying, recording or otherwise) without prior written permission of the author. Any person who does any unauthorised act in relation to this publication may be liable to criminal prosecution and civil claims for damages. Enquiries should be addressed to the publisher.

ISBN: 978-0-6488331-4-7

 A catalogue record for this book is available from the National Library of Australia

This book details the author's personal experiences with and opinions about perimenopause. The author is not a healthcare provider, and this book is not intended as a substitute for the medical advice of a licensed healthcare practitioner or physician. The statements made about products and services are not intended to diagnose, treat, cure, or prevent any condition or disease. Please consult with your own physician or healthcare specialist regarding any suggestions or recommendations made in this book. The reader should consult a physician in matters relating to their health and particularly with respect to any symptoms that may require diagnosis or medical attention. Neither the author or publisher, nor any contributors or other representatives, will be liable for damages arising out of or in connection with the use of this book. This is a comprehensive limitation of liability that applies to all damages of any kind, including (without limitation) compensatory; direct, indirect or consequential damages; loss of data, income or profit; loss of or damage to property and claims of third parties. This book is not intended as a substitute for consultation with a licensed healthcare practitioner, such as your physician.

Front cover design: Peter Morley, Good Catch Design
Back Cover Layout & Internal Design by Zena Shapter

Typeset in Palantino, Calibri Light and League Spartan

This book is dedicated to everyone* who had the misfortune of meeting me during my hormonal exodus.

It's likely I forgot your name, how I knew you, or what I was even doing there. I may or may not have been quarrelsome and annoying, I can't remember. I sweated and said f*ck a lot.

It wasn't me, it was my hormones.

———

*Especially Nick who suffered the most through my madness yet generously offered his hanky, his kindness and love. x

Contents

Foreword	9
by Dr. Angela Derosa, Do Mba Cpe Aka Dr. Hot Flash	
1. The Nuggets of Truth	11
2. Menopause. Kill Me Now	15
Common symptoms	16
What influences symptoms?	17
3. Be Prepared, Not Alarmed: My Story	19
4. Haywire Hormones	27
Oestrogen	28
Progesterone	30
Testosterone	31
Add thyroid into the mix	33
Your itinerary	36
5. HRT is not the Devil's Work	37
Origins	37
A note on gender bias	38
HRT controversy	39
HRT endorsed and supported by new findings	40
Compounded bioidentical hormone therapy	43
Tibolone	46
Another potential solution	47
My experience	48
Interlude – Important Information to Ponder	51

6. Not Just Vital for Boy Bands – Testosterone	55
One size does not fit all	57
A medical maze	58
Off-label prescriptions	60
The plot thickens	62
7. Alternatives to Hormone Therapies	67
Non-hormone prescription medications	67
Herbal therapies	70
Non-herbal therapies	72
Complementary therapies	73
Example: a naturopathic approach	73
Your body, your choice	74
8. Your Body Is a Temple	77
Tips for worshipping at the altar of your body	82
9. What to Take to Your Doctor	85
Firstly, what kind of doctor should you see?	85
Be prepared	86
10. Let's Embrace the Renewal Years	91
Acknowledgements	97
The Naked Truth About YOU	103

Foreword

by Dr. Angela DeRosa, DO MBA CPE aka Dr. Hot Flash

Perimenopause and menopause. How do two words evoke so much confusion and fear in both women and men alike? The truth behind the transition to menopause has been cloaked in mystery and poked fun at by comedians for far too long.

Hormone deficiencies are a serious matter and our mothers and grandmothers suffered in silence, often turning to wine or anti-anxiety medications to cope. But our current generation of mid-life women will not stay silent. We are finding a voice to tell it like it is.

In *The Naked Truth about PERIMENOPAUSE,* Susanne Mitchell takes an eye-opening look at this serious topic, her endearing sense of humor reading like an honest conversation with a well-informed girlfriend, while providing thought-provoking information and common sense advice. Susanne also offers context to 'conventional medical thinking', how to better approach potential 'conflicts of interest' in medicine and the very real gender biases we face in the treatment of women's hormonal health.

After going through an early menopause at age 35, I wish that I'd had some of these coping strategies, or the very least someone who could help me figure out what was happening to me. Menopause is the *'Elvis has left the building'* moment of our ovaries, but the exit is a slow process in most and we can take more than 10 years to get there. During this decade, women can have a whole variety of symptoms related to hormone decline that are often mislabeled as crazy, stressed or fibromyalgic. The more we talk about it out in the open, warts and all, the better we can care for ourselves and our fellow sisters in 'hot flashes'.

As a female doctor of internal medicine and hormonal specialist, I have found a kindred spirit in Susanne, as she provides women with much-needed information and coping strategies. I laughed, I cried, and I peed my pants a little when I read this book! I also got enraged once again, reading her struggle to understand and fight to access all the things that prevent women from getting the proper care and hormones they need. Men get their penis drugs and all the testosterone they require; we get psych meds and excuses.

Ultimately, hormone replacement therapy can treat the root cause of many of the disabling symptoms of hormone decline and menopause. It should not be feared, despite everything you hear in the media; but for those who want a broader understanding, or for women whom hormone therapy is not appropriate, this book is just what the doctor ordered.

1. The Nuggets of Truth

Remember when you went through puberty and the women in your life told you that you were about to become a woman? There was something all-knowing and slightly mysterious in their demeanour, like they knew stuff you didn't, but they weren't ever going to share it. When you head towards menopause, nobody tells you what you're going to become. They *allude* to it in whispered secret code, because female biology is classified information. Full disclosure might cause shame or serious injury to the national interest.

You keep calm and carry on, not expecting it to happen yet. Then suddenly you're hot, you're cold, your body begins to go through all this crazy shit, you're exhausted, you pile on weight and on top of all that, you begin to lose your mind. In a fit of anger, you consider running up the back of cars and stabbing your significant other.

I hear a lot of this partner-stabbing malarkey in menopause support groups on Facebook. Nobody tells you that you might one day become a murderer. It's those pesky hormones. Sorry, did I ovary act?

Recently, perimenopause hit me in all of its hot-flash, brain fog, hormonal glory as my body retreated into a chrysalis of transformation. I was unprepared and quite possibly in denial. If someone had shared the nuggets of truth within this book with me, then the last few years of my life would have made SO much more sense. Perhaps I wasn't prepared to listen. Menopause seemed very far away and anyway, I wasn't going to end up like that. No way.

And I repeated this to myself over the years, I turned 35, 40, 45, and 47. And when I turned 48 I was still knee-deep in denial, and yet I'd already begun the transition. I ended up in the depths of despair, behaving erratically as my hormones fled in a mass exodus. I'd had my oestrogen fix removed and didn't understand what that meant.

After wading through research, opinions, women's health forums and listening to medical professionals, I began to explore a range of lifestyle and medical options to help restore my state of balance. Eventually I found a route that brought me back to sanity.

Had I understood the process, perhaps I could have made better decisions to help me through. This is why I'm writing this for you. Perhaps I can spare you (or those who love you) some heartache. If you're reading this I'm guessing you're either knee-deep in perimenopause, or heading in that direction, or perhaps you're supporting your wife, partner, sister, or your mother through the unpredictable transition from a fertile to a non-reproductive state. Around half the population will go through this transformation and the rest may be affected by it directly at some point. Yet weirdly we mostly remain in the dark over the whole shebang, and rather worryingly it seems that so do many members of the medical profession. That's so wrong.

This stuff should not be a state secret, shrouded in conflict, whispers and myth. Let me reveal to you what I learned from personal experience and during my research for this book. I discovered that there's far more at play than you might think, especially when it comes to women's health.

Through this part of the adventure, I encountered eminent thought leaders and specialists in women's health, some of whom kindly gave me their time, opinion and expertise. After seeing two general practitioners, one in a specialist women's health clinic, I spoke directly with Michael Buckley, pharmacist, CEO and medical director of topical hormone cream manufacturer Lawley Pharmaceuticals. He shared his knowledge and looked at an early draft of the book.

I also took private consultation with Associate Professor John Eden, a gynaecologist and reproductive endocrinologist (a specialist in women's hormones) who has authored over 100 scientific papers and two books. Dr. Eden read an early draft of the book and set me straight on a few things from a medical perspective, as did Professor Susan Davis, a clinical researcher, specialist endocrinologist, president of the International Menopause Society and professor of Women's Health at Monash University. She has published more than 330 peer-reviewed manuscripts and has many professional associations to her name.

At this point, I took a breath to check my research and read more peer-reviewed academic papers, articles, reviews and studies. I'm not a doctor, I'm a creative professional, and so this work was demanding. I stressed and at times stared blankly at research papers, scratching my head to wonder what the hell I was doing. I knew there was more to it, because I'd found other, conflicting opinions; indeed my own experience conflicted with much of the evidence that had been presented.

> *"Difference of opinion leads to enquiry, and enquiry to truth; and that, I am sure, is the ultimate and sincere object of us both."*
>
> Thomas Jefferson 13th March 1815

But I couldn't find a way through the medical glass ceiling, so believing I had done my best, I quietly uploaded the book to Amazon prior to a publicity-and-book launch. One day later, hours before a meeting with my friend and publicist Valerie McIver, I received an email response, from a doctor, researcher and respected author of a paper I'd read back at the beginning.

And there it was: the glass ceiling cracked open enough for someone to reach out a hand to guide my enquiry further. I took the book down and entered months more research and rewrites. I had presentations and more papers, information on random control trials and observational studies. A whole new world opened up in my search for answers.

I entered into personal correspondence with Dr. Rebecca L. Glaser, MD, FACS, a retired breast cancer surgeon who is currently involved in research on testosterone therapy and its impact on health and breast cancer prevention. She's authored many peer-reviewed papers and also treats men and women with subcutaneous testosterone therapy.

And also with Dr. Angela DeRosa, DO, MBA, CPE, who specialises in women's hormonal health and has more than 25 years of experience in clinical practice. She shared her broad knowledge and time to review my work and write a foreword.

Opinions between our medical friends vary, but as Thomas Jefferson said to Peter H. Wendover, "Difference of opinion leads to enquiry, and enquiry to truth; and that, I am sure, is the ultimate and sincere object of us both."

My endeavour to find the truth about perimenopause and the best way through has been a challenging journey and one that continues to be a work in progress. There are always new scientific findings and roads ahead to explore, so I will keep you updated on the way. Together we can become informed, find solutions, get on with our lives and not just survive, but thrive. Let's go.

2. Menopause. Kill Me Now

Let's look behind the scenes at what menopause really means. Menopause is a catch-all term that lumps perimenopause, menopause and postmenopause into one. But menopause itself marks the permanent end of a woman's menstrual years, 12 months after her last period. It mostly occurs between the ages of 45–55. By the age of 54 around 80 percent of women have stopped having periods.[1]

Menopause is like the end titles rolling on a movie, the matriarchal moment after the drama that takes all the credit. It's a fleeting moment of 'thank f**k' before beginning *postmenopause*, where we emerge with altered biology from the chrysalis of *perimenopause*.

Prior to menopause, there are three major sex hormones circulating in a woman's blood: oestrogen, testosterone and progesterone. Unlike the sudden fall in oestrogen and progesterone at menopause, testosterone levels fall more gradually with increasing age.[2]

During the transformation of perimenopause, a woman's oestrogen levels fluctuate with erratic peaks and lows, inconsistent levels of progesterone are common and both cause wide-ranging changes in the menstrual cycle.[3] Unsurprisingly, the change of hormone levels causes our bodies to behave differently.[4] This hormonal chaos and rollercoaster retreat can feel like we are losing our minds and control of our emotions and bodily functions.

For some it can be an extremely long and tricky transition; others may cruise through with few symptoms.

The average time for perimenopause is four years,[5] but it can take longer for some women, and symptoms may appear as early as 10 years before the last period.[6] Although you may not link them to the process at this point, when you do, all that weirdness will suddenly make sense.

Common symptoms

Perimenopausal symptoms are why women in midlife were once committed to psych wards for hysteria. Like frenemies, they have a silent, ulterior motive to humiliate you, and they're the ones we need to understand and deal with before they steal away our confidence. I know. It sounds like midlife *Love Island*, doesn't it? But without the swaggering testosterone bluff and bravado. All the common symptoms are associated with a decrease of oestrogen:[7]

- hot flushes or flashes (same thing, I prefer flash, reminds me of a '70s disco)
- exhaustion, fatigue, night sweats, difficulty sleeping
- excessive bleeding, urge incontinence, dry vagina
- irritability, anger, mood swings,
- heart palpitations,[8] anxiety and an inability to cope with stress
- decreased cognitive function and memory fog, loss of confidence
- slower metabolism, joint pain and abdominal fat gain.[9]

Twenty-five per cent of women will have no perimenopausal symptoms and 75 per cent will have some. A quarter of those will have severe symptoms that negatively affect their daily life.[10] That's a lot of us at risk of road rage or murderous intent.

But seriously, symptoms can have a major impact on a woman's quality of life, affecting her mental health and ability to function. This can cause a knock-on effect and sometimes devastating consequences for her relationships, family and career. When I discussed these figures with Dr. Angela DeRosa, she told me she believes they are highly understated and that the majority of women struggle with perimenopausal symptoms (some worse than others), and the quality of life for those who do is significantly affected. My mental health was very rocky at times with grief and confusion over what was happening to me.

What influences symptoms?

Researchers suggest that lifestyle, diet, exercise, smoking, socio-economic variances and reproductive history all play a role in the hormone levels and symptoms women experience. Women's experience of the transition is also influenced by cultural attitudes and expectations.

In many parts of the world this transition is understood as a process, part of the phenomenon of aging, and is associated with both social and biological changes. It represents the beginning of freedom and new respect or status for women.

In North America, Europe and Australasia, we mostly think of menopause as the end of menstruation – a purely biological event. Most of us Westerners agree that perimenopause sucks. We don't see the rewards or positive changes because our society values youthful beauty over wisdom and wealth of experience. We feel pressured to stay looking young rather than embracing our laughter lines and grey hair.

Next up, we're going to look at my story to see how I got caught in the quicksand of perimenopausal chaos. And it's a precautionary tale. I was not ready. You can be way savvier than me.

3. Be Prepared, Not Alarmed: My Story

*A Girl Scout is ready to help out wherever she is needed.
Willingness to serve is not enough;
you must know how to do the job well,
even in an emergency.*

Girl Scout Handbook

I was once a Brownie, then a Girl Guide, but somehow, when it came to perimenopause, I'd forgotten our motto from back in the day: *Be Prepared*. I learned by bitter experience, but in my defence, I was a Brownie Guide like three minutes ago – deep in denial about my age and stage of life.

Now I've reflected, stumbled, done the research, seen how others have done well in their menopause journey, and am willing to serve up what I have learned. Knowledge, understanding the science, lifestyle, medical options and support from others are all key in navigating the best route.

Confucius said, 'By three methods we may learn wisdom: First, by reflection, which is noblest; Second, by imitation, which is easiest; and third by experience, which is the bitterest.' The third method is my experience.

In 2018 my daughter and I took my son on a once-in-a-lifetime special surprise 16th birthday trip to New York. We lived in Sydney, Australia, and I'd barely taken them on holidays, as money had always been tight.

On this much anticipated and planned adventure, I was hit with mood swings and a desperate sense of irrelevance. I should have been thrilled to witness my children in their element with their lives ahead of them, exploring an exciting new city.

But I lacked vitality, energy and my usual bright disposition. At 48 years old I felt strangely disenchanted, a sense of doom descending on me, an uncomfortable idea that my window of opportunity had passed me by. I considered that this might be IT, and quite frankly, IT wasn't enough.

Maybe I'd missed the boat of achieving my potential, doing unfulfilling work, knowing I had more to offer, but somehow failing to find or produce it.

Earlier that year I had suffered occasional hot flashes (also known as vasomotor symptoms) without realising what they were. I would walk around sweating saying, 'Is it hot in here?' while my kids rolled their eyes, telling me the evening breeze was cool through the apartment.

That summer in New York I was a hot mess, even in air-conditioning. I'd begun to experience a weak pelvic floor and a cough or sneeze meant clenching or damp knickers. Plus I felt like a tired old woman.

My hair and skin were dry, I had aching joints and walking anywhere hurt. My clothes were tight and I'd gained a little weight after 10 years of going to the gym and maintaining my fitness. I couldn't work out simple itineraries or plans and suffered anxiety and lots of tears that I tried to keep hidden. But my children's eyes are beady, and they saw my lack of physical resilience and moments of chaos. It confused us all.

Before this I'd been a woman in her element. Happy and bright, young at heart, fun and brave. This balmy New York summer my confidence jumped off the Empire State building and ditched to the sidewalk. I was a shadow of my former self.

Have you experienced this feeling?

When we returned home to a Sydney winter I seemed to rebalance, I went back to yoga and the gym and my mental health buoyed again.

Feeling normal again, I met and fell in love with my now partner. Life was good. Client work was busy, the kids were happy and I figured it was time to know where I was up to in my menstrual cycle. I'd worn a Mirena IUD for birth control for 12 years and as a result, I barely bled. It had been a brilliant hiatus from periods and some great freedom, but it also meant I had no idea if I was still menstruating.

I didn't understand what perimenopause was; I thought menopause was the big cheese and the thing to get myself through. I figured it would happen somewhere in my 50s, and that seemed a long way away.

Where are you in this cycle? Do you know where your body sits on a hormonal level?

I asked my gynaecologist to remove my IUD, and my new fella showed great compassion through what happened next, mopping up the mess with quiet kindness. He's pretty handy with the stain remover.

I bled like something out of a horror movie for six to eight weeks. Some days I would get out of bed with blood pouring down my legs. Add into the mix that I'm a Type 1 diabetic, that's the chronic type (my pancreas hasn't worked since I was 13 years old), and my blood sugars were ditching and raising as my hormones played havoc.

While rebalancing my diabetes and seeing my endocrinologist for help, I also changed to a socially conscious, smart, savvy male doctor.

He proved to be a brilliant advocate of looking at my case holistically and in helping keep my chronic disease managed.

Eventually the tidal wave of bleeding settled and I began to have periods again. Sigh. I know, it had been a while. But for the first time in years my body experienced normal cycles, and I knew that I hadn't passed through menopause.

Then some stress hit when I lost my main client just weeks before Christmas. I decided to take a work sabbatical, using my savings to invest in myself and write a book, The Naked Truth About YOU*, that had been on a backburner for years. So began a purposeful, empowering journey of fulfilling my potential.

I felt fairly balanced and completely in creative flow, words poured out of me alongside regular, heavy periods. Missing my IUD, I experienced a gradual creep of weight gain, but instead of cranking up my gym visits I started to let exercise slide. I felt tired all the time and put it down to workload.

Around the time I turned 49, I began to notice memory loss, more than the usual forgetting names. I found myself doing out-of-character things, missing a girls' night out despite talking to my friends about it only hours before. Leaving pans on the stove burning and not noticing until the apartment was full of smoke.

Some mornings I would walk around my home not knowing what I had been in search of or why. Like Dory from *Finding Nemo* with grey roots and no energy.

And I couldn't grasp simple concepts. One day someone asked me what the next chapter in the book I was writing was about and I couldn't find it in my brain. I was utterly vacant. (Interestingly, it was called 'Who the Hell Are You?') I looked like an idiot who didn't know

---

*https://www.susanne-mitchell.com/book/

what she was doing, let alone who she actually was. I was mortified at my seeming stupidity.

Have you suffered brain fog or memory loss more than normal?

I took my memory issues to the doctor as my aunty had suffered early onset dementia, and I was given a memory test. The first question was 'What year is it?' and I said '2020'. It was 2019. I managed the other questions, and it was labelled as stress.

Heading home I watched *Still Alice*, a true story about how a linguistics professor at Columbia, and her family, deal with her diagnosis of familial Alzheimer's disease at age 50. I wallowed in self-pity and concern for myself while eating Cheezos, weeping and drinking wine. My poor brain function was terrifying.

As the year progressed, I tired more easily and figured it was the five- and six-day-weeks I was putting in on the book, long days of focused concentration. I was in and out of the doctor's surgery with memory-related problems, fatigue, anxiety, diabetes balance issues and weight-gain questions. We did blood tests for everything including thyroid, they all looked normal, but I was a mess. A puddle of doubt in hormonal free-fall.

I had regular periods until June, then July no bleeding and in August I bled lightly. September came and went, I bought bigger clothes for a second time that year. That combined with my inability to hold my own in conversations and my forgetfulness made me lose even more confidence.

> *'We did blood tests for everything including thyroid, they all looked normal but I was a mess. A puddle of doubt in hormonal free-fall.'*

I used to walk into rooms like I owned them, I felt comfortable in my skin and loved socialising and chatting with people. But suddenly I felt like an empty shell. With a sagging jawline, bulging muffin top and dinner lady arms my feminine power fled my once-defined waistline and took exile on my arse.

I had to think very deeply to focus on anything, and simple tasks took me forever. Some days I was so dog tired that I'd sit in my car trying to summon the strength to open the door. Then I'd need to rest at the front door. The stairs would loom ahead of me like Mount Everest: I could barely lift my legs to take the first step, let alone conquer the first floor.

Do you struggle to find energy to do everyday things?

My moods swung with regularity. I'd be bright then low then bright then low. Some days I just took myself to bed, and the low days hit me more and more regularly. And I was quick to lose my temper, I started to kick out at those I loved. I was becoming a right royal pain in the arse, and I knew it, I could see it, but I could not for the life of me stop it.

I went back to the doctor again and he checked for other chronic diseases like Coeliac. (If you have one autoimmune disease it's common to suffer another.) That thought sent me pretty darned blue; it's bad enough to manage Type 1 diabetes with a life-saving insulin pump attached 24/7, let alone having to consider another autoimmune disease.

Some days I felt desperately low with grief and confusion over losing myself and managing a body that seemed to be falling apart. I also have a frozen shoulder, and the pain and lack of mobility made me cranky and sore. I wasn't sleeping. And I hadn't really considered that my periods had stopped. Perhaps that was the brain fog. By this point, if I hadn't had my kids, good friends or my loving partner, I might not have made it through.

'With a sagging jawline, bulging muffin top and dinner lady arms my feminine power fled my once defined waistline and took exile on my arse.'

Is it me or is it hot in here?

Then the hot flashes started. A few times a day I would be hit out of nowhere with a rush of heat from my feet to the tips of my ears. No discrimination – it would happen in the middle of a meeting, driving, at the supermarket checkout – they blazed through me like bushfires.

Quickly I found myself having one every waking hour and then night sweats that saw me kicking off covers and switching on fans, driving my man mad. Exhausted and beyond ok with it all, I could see the strain it had put on our relationship.

Have you burned up with hot flashes?

I started to read about hot flashes and menopause. Rather belatedly I made the connection between my poor brain function, exhaustion, short temper, poor skin and hair, painful joints, leaky sneezes and night sweats and flashes. I had been quite confused and grumpy for some time and very slow to be aware of the cause. Sounds ridiculous, I know.

Then I began to talk to other women of my age. Some randomly at the supermarket or in the pharmacy when a flash hit me. And many sympathised or shared their stories, talking in whispers with eyes rolling.

A covert club

It was like a secret society cracked open its door to me and I wrenched it open, so angry it hadn't allowed me access earlier. I was mad as a cut snake. I'd been through hell for 18 months and thought I was losing my mind. All the while other women were also suffering in silence.

With the exhaustion and memory fog becoming increasingly debilitating, I started to read up on perimenopause. I joined Facebook groups and read articles by professionals specialising in menopause. Blood tests had shown my hormones were running screaming to the hills, and I began to look at what that meant and what options I had to help me cope. I started to educate myself over natural therapies and hormone replacement therapy (HRT), which is now also known as menopausal hormone treatment (MHT) – they are the same thing.

I began to wonder why we don't replace the testosterone we've lost alongside the female reproductive hormones when using HRT? This didn't make sense to me.

Just before Christmas 2019, hot flashes raged through me a couple of times an hour, sweat ran down my back and I felt out of control and desperate for help. My brain misfired constantly over simple things adding confusion and frustration into the mix. I had no energy, no light, I wasn't sleeping through night sweats and my emotions were frayed. The Susanne I once knew seemed like a distant memory.

My life had become a living hell. If an asylum had been closer than my doctor's surgery I would have handed myself in. But it wasn't. My doctor made the call that I needed HRT to get balance back and keep me from being bound in a straightjacket. I was exhaustipated; I couldn't have given a shit what was suggested, I would have taken it to feel normal again. *Anything* to feel normal.

> *'Hot flashes raged through me every hour, sweat ran down my back and I felt out of control and desperate for help.'*

I was so far away from my Brownie Guide motto, I had never been so unprepared in my life. Here's what I wish I'd understood before the big transformation.

4. Haywire Hormones

When your hormones go haywire they become horrormones. When we first experience their full-force through our teenage years we may suffer pimples and protrusions and sometime smell like off-cheese, but opportunities await us and the world is at our feet. Plus we know everything.

During your fertile years you're up, you're down, you bleed and you're like, 'I love you, I hate you, I'm sorry it's my period, I'm hormonal so if you aren't coffee, chocolate, wine or Cheezos I'm going to need you to f*ck off.' You think 'I'll get to menopause and *all of this* will go away.' Then your hormones pack up and run off with your period and you're *still*, 'I love you, I hate you, I'm sorry, I've forgotten what I'm doing in here, when did I get so fat and who the hell am I?' It's like they ditch the party but leave behind their bad '80s shoulder pads and mood swings. It starts to dawn on us that we don't know everything after all.

Women's ovaries produce oestrogen, progesterone and testosterone, and in addition to this the adrenal glands produce a hormone called DHEA, which can be used by the ovaries and other cells in the body to make oestrogens and testosterone.[11] Our thyroid is also worth noting here as thyroid hormones fuel and control your metabolism.[12]

Dr. Angela DeRosa specialises in women's hormonal health, spending 10 years as a medical director with a large pharmaceutical company in her early career, and she has more than 25 years' experience in clinical practice. She's seen hormone deficiency from all angles: as a patient who suffered early menopause at 35-years-old, as a doctor at her Hormonal Health Institute, from Big Pharma's perspective and now as a medical director with Belmar, a large compounding pharmaceutical company. It's a very unique perspective.

She believes that women are getting bad information about hormones and hormone replacement therapies from their doctors, the media and government, and that's causing a health epidemic.[13] Hormone deficiency can be debilitating and cause a devastating domino effect on our personal and working relationships.

Add to that, says Dr. DeRosa, deficiency in thyroid hormones, oestrogen, testosterone, vitamin D (yes, it's a hormone!) all lead to inflammatory states that increase the risk of cancer. And they predispose women (and men) to chronic illness.

Without hormones we wouldn't grow, have libidos or reproduce; they are essential in leading a balanced life. Produced by the endocrine system, these chemical messengers send commands around the body helping to regulate your body's processes, like hunger, blood pressure and sexual desire.

> *'I love you, I hate you, I'm sorry, I've forgotten what I'm doing in here, when did I get so fat and who the hell am I?'*

Basically hormones tell your body how to breathe, grow, drink, eat and expend energy. They are your inner dominatrix, you are their submissive. Let's take a look at the all-important sex-hormones.

Oestrogen

Both sexes produce oestrogen, and women make three types: estriol, which is largely produced during pregnancy; estrone, which can be toxic and inflammatory and is made in our fat from estradiol; and estradiol, which is the Fairy Godmother of the three.[14]

In females oestrogen is responsible for:

- sexual development on reaching puberty
- managing the growth of the uterine lining, causing breast changes in teenagers and pregnant women
- bone and cholesterol metabolism
- protecting bone health (in men too)
- affecting your brain (including mood), heart, skin, and other tissues[15]
- regulating food intake, body weight, glucose metabolism, and insulin sensitivity.

The female hormone oestrogen can sometimes stimulate breast cancer cells and cause them to grow. Women who are obese will produce more estrone from fatty tissue. Too much estrone (the bad one that's made in our fat) has been linked to breast and endometrial cancer growth. Besides this potential outcome, other results of increased estrone levels are not yet known.[16]

Lowered levels of oestrogen after menopause can lead to troublesome postmenopausal symptoms.[17] Typical symptoms of low oestrogen are painful sex due to a lack of vaginal lubrication, increased urinary tract infections, irregular periods, mood swings, hot flashes, breast tenderness, headaches, anxiety, depression, joint pain, trouble concentrating and fatigue.[18] So basically everything.

During the early stages of perimenopause as oestrogen declines, many women may experience hot flashes and insomnia just before their period. Premenstrual syndrome (PMS) can get worse and migraines may appear. Through the mid-stage of oestrogen deficiency, hot flashes burn through at random times in the month, PMS can crank up alongside insomnia, forgetfulness and night sweats. The late stage sees a worsening of overall symptoms and irregularity in menstrual cycles.[19]

Oestrogen deficiency also leads to a hardening of the arteries, which causes high blood pressure and increases LDL (bad cholesterol) and lowers HDL (good cholesterol), which can lead to heart disease.[20]

Decreasing oestrogen can also lead to bone loss and an increased risk of fragility fractures[21]. Osteoporosis is very common among women and is known as the silent killer. An absence of symptoms doesn't mean bone loss and other metabolic changes aren't occurring. Women experience a rapid decline in bone density after menopause when the ovaries stop producing oestrogens, and oestrogen levels are considered to be some of the strongest risk factors for osteoporosis.[22]

> *'Most of my pantry seems to be stored in the fat on my arse since my oestrogen stores ran out.'*

Progesterone

Both sexes produce progesterone, but men only have a small amount to help with sperm development. In women it:

- helps regulate the menstrual cycle
- helps thicken the lining of the uterus after monthly ovulation to prepare for a fertilised egg
- helps maintain the uterus lining if a woman becomes pregnant
- is necessary for breast development and breast feeding.

Low progesterone can cause irregular periods, abnormal bleeding, mood changes, headaches or migraines and difficulty in getting or staying pregnant. Without progesterone to compensate it, oestrogen may become the dominant hormone. If a woman doesn't ovulate, her ovaries don't produce progesterone.[23]

Progesterone is produced when the egg is released at ovulation, and it controls the growth of the uterine lining (endometrium). Menstrual periods can become heavier and more problematic during the perimenopausal transition due to too much oestrogen and not enough progesterone.[24]

Progesterone in the bioidentical form, or the synthetic progestogen, are used together with oestrogen in hormone replacement therapy (HRT, also known as menopause hormone therapy, MHT) because oestrogen causes the lining of the uterus to thicken. A thickened uterus lining may undergo cellular changes that have the potential to develop into uterine cancer.[25] When taking progesterone or progestogen for menopausal symptoms, side effects may include mood changes, bloating, headaches, and breast tenderness.[26] So what's new?

A note here about bioidentical and synthetic – more on this later in the HRT chapter – but avoid a synthetic progestogen or oestrogen if you can afford to.[27] Synthetic hormones look similar but have slightly altered chemistry, as this allows drug companies to patent the product. To do that they must change the chemical structure (risking side effects) or offer a unique delivery method of the original molecule. Which would you rather take: something that has been adapted to make a profit or something identical to the natural hormone?[28]

Testosterone

> *'I'm not talking about testosterone as in 25-year-old boyfriends, but in the form of a hormone cream that's harder to score than heroin.'*

Testosterone is made in men's testes and women's ovaries. It's also produced in the adrenal glands in both sexes. Testosterone and other related hormones in the body (also known as androgens) have important roles in healthy women. It is generally known that testosterone is important for muscle and bone strength and for growth of normal body hair. But testosterone may have favourable effects on mood, wellbeing, energy and 'vitality' in women.[29]

Studies have shown improvements in various aspects of female sexuality with testosterone therapy. Other research claims that testosterone plays a critical role in both sexes, and the benefits of testosterone therapy go well beyond sex drive and libido, to aiding the brain and nervous system, affecting our skin, cardiovascular system and other essential organs.[30] Testosterone is essential for glucose metabolism and maintaining weight. Who doesn't want that? And it's the most abundant biologically active hormone in women's bodies.[31]

Testosterone will usually start to decline before oestrogen and is deficient for longer, given that we lose our oestrogen later and Mother Nature stores it in our fat. Most of my pantry seems to be stored in the fat on my arse since my oestrogen stores ran out! A deficiency in testosterone also causes risk for pre-diabetes, type 2 diabetes, heart disease and osteoporosis.[32]

"If you were to put a gun to my head, I'd choose testosterone over oestrogen, although hot flashes and night sweats (as well as other symptoms of estrogen deficiency) suck, testosterone deficiency is much more impactful. When deficient, women start to develop mood disorders (depression, anxiety, panic attacks), impaired cognition, migraine headaches, weight gain and all the cardiovascular risks that follow, as well as inflammation, which puts women at risk of cancer, including breast cancer. And let's not forget that testosterone deficiency also leads to the death of our sexual being, which then predisposes us to relationship problems," says Dr. DeRosa.

A former breast cancer surgeon, Dr. Rebecca Glaser, is involved in research on testosterone therapy and its impact on health and breast cancer prevention. She refutes many of the myths and misconceptions that currently exist around testosterone therapy in women and agrees that testosterone is essential for both our physical and mental health.[33] Dr. Glaser is an assistant clinical professor at Wright State University in Ohio and has authored many peer reviewed papers on testosterone therapy.

When fully functioning, a woman's body makes 60 percent oestrogen and 40 percent testosterone; a man makes 95 percent testosterone and five percent oestrogen. In either sex, if testosterone levels become imbalanced, adverse symptoms such as the following can occur:

- decreased sex drive
- lack of motivation, anxiety, depression
- difficulty concentrating and memory loss
- sugar craving, weight gain – particularly in the belly.[34]

I've devoted a chapter to testosterone later in this book because of the importance of androgens in our bodies and their effect on our health and wellbeing. And I'm not talking about testosterone as in 25-year-old boyfriends, but in the form of a hormone cream that's harder to score than heroin.

Using testosterone to treat perimenopausal symptoms is controversial and the cause of much heated debate among medical professionals. It may also be influenced by pharmaceutical companies. I will expand on the commercial, political and often contentious side of medicine later in the book. Testosterone helped me to clear my brain fog and make it up the stairs again.[35]

Add thyroid into the mix

The thyroid gland plays a major role in the metabolism, growth and development of the human body. It helps to regulate many bodily functions by constantly releasing a steady amount of thyroid hormones into the bloodstream. If we suddenly need more energy – for instance, if we are growing or cold, or during pregnancy – the thyroid gland produces more hormones.[36]

Dr. Angela DeRosa believes thyroid hormones are the other important hormones at play, alongside oestrogen and testosterone. She says the thyroid is like the engine of our bodies; we don't want it to run too fast or slow, hot or cold, but to cruise along evenly.

"Women with normal thyroid function have appropriate energy levels and feel good, assuming they have no other health issues," says Dr. DeRosa. "But by the age of 50, one in three women will have a thyroid disorder; most commonly they'll be hypothyroid, or low thyroid. Thyroid deficiency leads to cholesterol issues, which leads to heart disease and these are just a few examples."

An underactive thyroid (hypothyroid) or slow running engine can cause:

- fatigue, weight gain, muscle aches, slow heart rate
- intolerance to cold, constipation, hair loss, dry skin
- irritability, depression, memory loss.

An overactive thyroid (hyperthyroid) or fast running engine can cause:

- fatigue, difficulty sleeping or weight loss
- intolerance to heat, excessive sweating, diarrhoea or itching
- nervousness, anxiety, high blood pressure, rapid or irregular pulse.[37]

Combine low oestrogen, testosterone and hypothyroidism, and that's a recipe for disaster. I honestly had no idea how important a role our hormones play in our lives. I took them for granted when they were balanced. But when they went into freefall I had to scrabble and fight like hell to find the ripcord to survive and cope with life. Everything ditches with them.

It's an individual thing

Some people are more sensitive to hormones than others, which is why some women suffer premenstrual syndrome (PMS) or postpartum depression (PND) – when oestrogen levels plummet after giving birth. Or why some of us suffer through perimenopause and others barely notice it, cruising obliviously right on through and wondering what all the fuss is about.

Clearly I am super sensitive to the little blighters, although I didn't suffer difficult PMS, I did suffer PND. We are different. We are all beautiful. You are unique. I know. My eyes are in way better shape than the rest of me because I roll them like 386 times a day, mostly at myself.

Your itinerary

If your hormones are beginning to pack their bags then it's time to consider how you will manage that transition. And until you're in it, you don't know how it's going to play out for you. So getting prepared and educated will only see you make more informed decisions and help you stay afloat if you hit tumultuous seas.

Perhaps you'll want to check out natural therapies first. Or decide if hormone replacement is worth exploring. One solution will not fit all. Do your own research and make sure you're giving yourself the best chance to retain your sanity, health and relationships. Let's keep the rage off the roads and partners safe from sharp implements.

5. HRT is not the Devil's Work

Hormone replacement therapy (HRT) or menopausal hormone treatment for women is medication that replaces oestrogen, progesterone and far more rarely, testosterone. It's prescribed in various combinations of pills, creams, gel, patches, IUDs and bioidentical pellets placed under the skin. The purpose of HRT is to manage the symptoms of menopause and improve quality of life. Doctors assess how to combine and apply the right combination according to your age and stage of menopause, taking risk factors into account.

HRT continues to be feared by women, despite about-turns and retractions of the way trial findings were initially communicated, all of which have received little publicity in the media compared to the initial furore. So many women have been influenced and misinformed by inflammatory and distorted breast cancer headlines. But this certainly isn't the whole story. Let's take a look at the history.

Origins

HRT was first available as an oestrogen pill in the 1940s, but became more widely used in the 1960s. Hormone therapy was marketed (mostly by men) as a way for women to end the curse of oestrogen loss, preserve femininity and stay young (for the benefit of keeping their men interested).

In 1966 Dr Robert Wilson's book *Feminine Forever*[38]'maintained that menopause was an estrogen-deficiency disease that should be treated with oestrogen replacement therapy to prevent the otherwise inevitable "living decay".'[39]

'All post-menopausal women are castrates,' Wilson wrote as he opined the 'tragedy of menopause' while feeding his patients 'youth pills'.[40] Some women embraced his ideas, others reeled at his misogyny. Now, 54 years on, I'm a feminist but I take HRT. Not to keep myself bathed in a mythical fountain of youth, but to take back control of my mental and physical wellbeing.

In the 1970s it was found that oestrogen supplements were associated with an increased risk of endometrial cancer. This had a bad impact on HRT's reputation, but then researchers discovered that reducing the dosage of estrogen and combining it with progesterone could reduce the risk of endometrial cancer. Such combined therapy was recommended for women with an intact uterus, raising renewed enthusiasm for HRT treatment which increased through the 1980s and '90s.[41]

The feminist discussion of menopause through this period revealed a larger agenda, that women should retain control of their bodies and participate fully in the decision-making efforts regarding their health. By controlling their bodies, all women, whether feminist or not, could ultimately control their lives.[42]

A note on gender bias

Disappointingly, women continue to experience a gender bias in both our culture and in medicine. For example, women with endometriosis in Australia commonly have to seek second, third, and even further opinions from different doctors before they find one who takes their complaints seriously, diagnoses them accurately, and treats them effectively.[43]

In 2018 a ten-year-study published in the British Heart Association journal found that more than 8,200 women in England and Wales could have survived their heart attacks had they simply been given the same quality of treatment as men.[44]

In the USA there's an overwhelming number of men (and women) in government who want to legislate control of women's bodies. It is madness that we are still having the same arguments about contraception and reproductive healthcare for women, the same arguments that we had in the 1960s and 70s and for decades before that time.[45]

HRT controversy

In 1991 the Women's Health Initiative (WHI) began a study of 162,000 women to find out if older women who started on HRT *after* menopause would get the same benefits to their heart-health as younger women who started HRT during perimenopause. (The treatment was not the safer transdermal oestrogen and micronised progesterone that would be used today.)

But the WHI trial was designed to focus on long-term hormone therapy to prevent chronic disease in women over 60, and only 30 per cent of the study participants were aged 50 to 59 (the years in which most women undergo HRT). The results were generalised to these younger women on short-term therapy for symptoms of menopause.[46]

A second initiative, the Million Women Study which reviewed women booked in for a mammogram and was not a randomised trial, began in 1996. Reported results from both studies raised concerns regarding the safety of HRT.

These safety concerns revolved around two main issues:
- that the extended use of HRT may increase the risk of breast cancer, and
- that the use of HRT may increase the risk of heart disease.

In 2002 an initial results paper of the WHI study and premature press release – written in secret by a small group of the study executives – cited an increase in breast cancer as the main reason for terminating the trial. It also cited an increase in heart attacks.[47] This frightening information was leaked days before the full study was published, and the media fanned the flames with sensational headlines.

The medical profession was forced to field the hysteria that ensued without access to the results of the study. As a result, many women immediately stopped taking HRT, and that interpretation has since gained wide and uncritical acceptance.[48]

This ultimately caused substantial and ongoing harm to a generation of women for whom appropriate and beneficial treatment was either cut short or never started.

But on later investigation the study results were not statistically significant for breast cancer harm. They showed the younger women aged 50 to 59 had less than a third of a risk than the women aged 70 to 79. Plus the results weren't adjusted for factors such as pre-existing diseases or other treatments.[49] According to Robert Langer, who was involved in early leadership of the study, the trial was terminated early based on a finding of likely futility, not harm.[50]

The Million Women Study results were critically reviewed by Professor Sam Shapiro in 2004. He found that the study contained multiple errors and that the conclusion that it has been established that hormone therapy increases the risk of breast cancer was not justified.[51]

HRT endorsed and supported by new findings

Over recent years consideration of further research has led to a recognition that for most women who begin HRT under the age of 60 (or within ten years of menopause), HRT provides more benefits than risks.[52]

In 2015 the National Institute for Health and Clinical Excellence (UK) said millions of women should no longer have to suffer in silence; HRT worked, it said. When the data was re-examined for women who started HRT during menopause, it showed *no increased risk of breast cancer*. The increased risk was only associated with women who started taking HRT long after menopause.

In 2017 the WHI published its long-term findings concluding that women do not die from taking HRT. Breast cancer risks were not high, with the WHI study putting it at one *more* case in 1000. Haitham Hamoda, consultant gynaecologist at Kings College Hospital and spokesman for the Royal College of Obstetricians and Gynaecologists, stated that one in 1000 'in medical and statistical terms is a small number. It is similar to the [breast cancer] risk of drinking a glass of wine a night.' The risk of breast cancer from being overweight is four times higher.[53]

The study found that if women start HRT around the time of menopause the risk is very small, but only limited data was available for continued usage beyond the age of 60. The balance of benefit to harm always needs to be assessed, but appears to have shifted favourably for HRT.[54]

Other studies have found that HRT protects the bones and heart and may help women's memory.[55] This is important if periods stop very early and a factor to consider at the average menopause age.

A large controlled trial from Denmark in 2012 reported that healthy women taking combined HRT for 10 years immediately after menopause had a reduced risk of heart disease and of dying from heart disease.[56]

Despite all of these studies, there remains widespread distrust, confusion and uncertainty among doctors and the general community. Dr JoAnn Manson says that care for midlife women is still 'quite fragmented and derailed'. Many doctors are reluctant or lack the training to prescribe appropriate hormone therapy, she says. At the same time, there's been an explosion in the market for unproven alternative treatments.[57]

In 2013 a study was published that estimated between 2002 and 2012 as many as 19,610 postmenopausal American women died prematurely as a result of avoiding oestrogen therapy.[58]

We are all different

Most medications carry risks and for some women – like those at high risk of breast or ovarian cancer – those risks *are* too high. Every woman is different, and it's important you or the peri-woman in your life discuss individual needs with your healthcare provider. If you aren't being heard by them (which happens too often), then find a specialist in hormones or women's health. See Chapter 9 for more ideas on this. There are no easy answers, so be prepared to lobby for the healthcare you deserve.

For many women HRT is a life-saver, and society must respect your right to choose what will work best for you. If you want to read in more detail you'll find more resources at the end of this book.

Dr. DeRosa is vocal about the importance of hormone therapy in both sexes, but she is particularly passionate about helping women, because she says we still don't have a voice in medicine. "We are excluded from research trials, because they're afraid we might get pregnant, that the baby may be affected, and the liability is way too high. So there's a tremendous gender bias in research trials, and as a result women don't get an equal voice or respect when it comes to their unique medical needs, in particular with regards to their hormones. They frankly get screwed."

Compounded bioidentical hormone therapy

Compounded bioidentical menopausal hormone therapies are various hormonal preparations aimed at correcting hormonal imbalances. Women turned to compounded bioidentical therapies following the HRT hysteria of 2002 as they sought alternative treatments to manage their menopausal symptoms. These compounds can contain a combination of oestrogens, progesterone and other hormonal compounds such as DHEA, testosterone, and melatonin.[59]

Being based on the unique idiosyncratic nature of each individual patient, compounded bioidentical therapies can allow more tailored therapies in varying formulations, if you suffer an allergy to ingredients in a commercial product, for example. There are pellets, topical gels, creams, soluble tablets, fast burst sublinguals, powder, troches (lozenges) and vaginal creams.

Compounding accounted for 80 percent of prescriptions until the second half of the 20th century, when the mass production of drugs began to dominate the mainstream market, moving pharmaceutical preparation from a pharmacy context to a manufacturing one. Today, more than 90 percent of medicinal products are industrial but regardless, many patients with particular needs depend on this important therapeutic service.[60]

Pharmaceutical companies cannot secure a patent (a legally enforceable right to commercially exploit the invention) on a bio-identical molecule like oestrogen or testosterone. Not unless it has something unique about it, such as a special delivery system, like a patch for example.

The term 'bioidentical' has been defined by the Endocrine Society as 'compounds that have exactly the same chemical and molecular structure as hormones that are produced in the human body'. The term 'body-identical' is used interchangeably. Some prescribed HRT is 'bioidentical' and some is not.[61]

Commercial hormone products that aren't bioidentical are a synthetic derivative that look similar but have other chains of chemistry, so they are altered slightly. To be clear, both types are made in the laboratory with differing chemistry.

Synthetic hormones delivered via a pill may be dangerous (or at the very least don't work as well) for women. Because pills process in the digestive system, then, when they metabolise in the liver before entering the blood stream, the hormone metabolism can cause the liver to kick out clotting factors. These clotting factors then increase the risk of developing deep vein thrombosis, pulmonary embolism, strokes and heart attacks.[62]

There are however some good quality bioidentical products such as Prometrium, a progesterone gel capsule[63] which can be taken orally or vaginally, Vivelle-Dot patches, Estrace cream and EstroGel for oestrogen replacement.

Okay, so this is where we open up a whole debate and opposing opinions in the medical profession. In Australia, the Royal Australian College of General Practitioners reports that compounded hormones are not required to undergo rigorous pharmaceutical and TGA testing. They state that there can be large variability in the concentrations of active and inactive ingredients, hence their efficacy is variable.[64]

Yet these therapies are prepared by trained pharmacists working to a specific prescription issued by a physician. The Pharmacy Board of Australia offers guidelines on the compounding of medicines for pharmacists, which are published on its website*. The dosage is formulated and compounded to meet the specific needs of each

---

*https://www.pharmacyboard.gov.au/codes-guidelines.aspx

patient, because one size does not fit all.[65] I reckon we can all relate to that!

In the UK, compounding pharmacies are regulated by and comply with the standards of the General Pharmaceutical Council (GPhC).[66]

In the USA there are two types of compounding pharmacy: the 503As, which are smaller and less highly regulated, and can give the industry a bad name if they don't adhere to the highest quality. Or there are the 503Bs, which are highly regulated and routinely inspected by the U.S. Food and Drug Administration (FDA) or the Drug Enforcement Administration (DEA). These 503Bs must use base products that are FDA approved.[67]

The Australian Medical Society (AMS) does not endorse prescribing compounded bioidentical hormones, which leaves many doctors only prescribing big pharma products to patients. Are we lacking in training and the education of our healthcare providers in women's hormonal health? Do drug companies unduly influence our doctors in what they prescribe? Is it possible they influence the medical societies that we rely on for truthful reporting?

The Australian Menopause Society states on its website, 'In the absence of peer-reviewed scientific data, and for all the other reasons mentioned below, the Australasian Menopause Society cannot endorse the use of compounded bioidentical hormone therapies.' You can check out those reasons in their fact* sheet and make your own decision on treatment.

It's important to understand that compounded bioidentical hormones fill a void that is clearly not being met by commercial products for women. For example, testosterone is not available for women commercially outside Australia (and one product has only just received approval for

*https://www.menopause.org.au/hp/information-sheets/212-bioidentical-hormones-for-menopausal-symptoms

registration across Australia for a specific use – I'll explain more about this in the next chapter), but this vitally important hormone is available through compounding pharmacies throughout the world.

In the USA, the FDA has issued statements warning against the practice of prescribing non-FDA approved drugs.[68] Big pharmaceutical companies make massive profits selling their patented brand name drugs for high cholesterol, stress, sleep disorders, migraines, depression, type 2 diabetes, etc.

Dr. DeRosa says that all the symptoms these highly profitable drugs are designed to treat are most often related to hormone deficiencies. So most doctors are treating the symptoms and not the cause. Using HRT to effectively treat underlying hormone deficiencies in women can relieve symptoms and eliminate the need for most or all of those medications in most patients.[69] This would mean a huge drop in drug company profits.

"Lobbyists for the pharmaceutical industry are paid big bucks trying to kill access to non-patentable bioidentical hormones and they continue to circulate bad information about HRT to do it," she says. "Some big pharma companies are working overtime trying to shut down compounding pharmacies, insisting that doctors only be allowed to prescribe FDA-approved drugs (in other words drugs developed, promoted and profited on by big pharma.) If they succeed in their mission it will be devastating for women."[70]

We must demand the right to have a choice and variety of therapies available to us so that we can choose what is appropriate on an individual level.

Tibolone

Tibolone is a synthetic steroid molecule, derived from the Mexican yam, and is different from other HRT. Instead of actual hormones (such as oestrogen and progestogen) it contains tibolone, which has oestrogenic, androgenic and progestogenic effects. It's like tibolone cons you into the same effects and benefits as regular HRT. Your body breaks it down to make hormones.[71]

It is suitable for women who have passed menopause because if taken prior it can cause irregular bleeding.[72] Tibolone may interfere with the effectiveness of breast cancer therapies and its use is contraindicated in women with breast cancer.[73] It is thought to enhance testosterone availability by reducing sex hormone binding globulin (SHBG)[74] but the response to it is variable.[75] Phew! That science almost gave me a hot flash!

Another potential solution

Trials are underway for a new class of experimental drugs that target receptors in the brain and may provide hope for women who can't or don't want to use HRT. These drugs have been shown to reduce hot flashes by almost three-quarters in just three days and are thought to work by blocking the action of a brain chemical called neurokinin B (NKB). Previous animal and human trials have shown increased levels of NKB may trigger hot flashes.

An initial compound thought to prevent NKB activating temperature control areas in the brain was tested by scientists at Imperial College London. That compound also revealed sleep and concentration was significantly improved in the three-day window. Due to side effects that may affect liver function the compound wasn't taken further in trials.[76]

However, the good news is that two very similar drugs, which also block NKB but do not appear to carry these side effects, have entered larger patient trials, with one such trial launched in the US back in 2017. I'm looking forward to hearing those results.

My experience

My family doctor started me on combined HRT, he initially prescribed a synthetic oral progesterone and advised that using a transdermal oestrogen gel (which is rubbed into the skin) was a safer option than a pill as it has less effect on blood clotting. Taking oestrogen on its own can increase the risk of developing womb cancer and so during my first year of HRT, progesterone was used for 12 days of the month (cyclical) to help protect the lining of my womb. This meant that I bled after the 12 days of progesterone, that was the downside, I had my periods back for a while. Another option was to put the IUD back in through that first year (and into postmenopause) as this provides the protective progesterone *and* stops the monthly bleeding. I opted not to do that.

Once I had taken HRT for a year, or a year passed since my last menstrual period (Yay! – that moment of meno-pause – it happened recently) my doctor swapped me onto continual HRT by taking the progesterone daily. Now I rarely bleed, although I get some random breakthrough here and there.

Occasionally women raise their eyebrows at me for using HRT, because the myths persist out there. If they 'kept calm and carried on' this tells me that their symptoms were manageable and not sending them to the asylum. And I know others who have suffered debilitating symptoms well into their 60s because of the frightening results of those studies back in 2002/2003. I chose to save my sanity and my perimenopausal arse and reserve the right to change my mind about hormone therapy as I evolve. Many women find it works really well and others don't. The benefits for me, for the moment, outweigh the risks.

The relief from HRT started to kick in for me at around 2–3 weeks of use; my emotions became more balanced and the flushes were reduced significantly within the first week. Although it wasn't all just miraculously ok, I still suffered awful memory fog and fatigue.

A suspicion that low levels of testosterone might hold the key to my loss of brain function and energy grew with my research. After the interlude, I'll tell you what I discovered.

Interlude – Important Information to Ponder

Before heading into the next chapter, we need to consider this slight detour around perimenopause: that our physicians and the public at large rely on doctors, who are experts in specific areas of medicine, and on medical journals and societies, which we assume provide unbiased independent medical literature and information. This is a lofty or sugar-coated ideal but as we know, as nothing tastes that sweet and all good stories have deeper, sometimes bitter tasting plots of intrigue.

There are, and always will be conflicts of interest in the narrative of medicine or indeed life, for we all need to fund our basic needs. Let's define some of the roles in this play.

Doctors are most interested in patient care and scientific advance, while industry is way more interested in the bottom line and commercial outcomes. In patient care, the principal leading role is the patient, whereas the leading role for industry is the shareholder. The similarities and differences between the needs and interests of the leading protagonists creates both a need for discourse and the potential for conflict. The overriding plot line should be a firm belief that the values of science and clinical medicine must prevail over commercial imperatives.[77]

Enter stage right the hero, a cape-wearing physician and an expert in their field, often with impressive academic appointments; they are highly sought after by pharmaceutical companies to consult with them as a 'key opinion leaders' (KOL) or thought leaders.

They will give lectures or conduct clinical trials, and occasionally make presentations on behalf of big pharma at regulatory meetings or hearings.[78] Like an Instagram influencer on social media, they are effective at transmitting messages to their medical peer group.

These thought leaders don't obviously endorse drug products, but their opinions can be used to market them, via lectures, sponsored symposia, or articles in medical journals or for medical societies (which may be ghostwritten by hired medical writers). They may take the money, status, and perks that pharmaceutical companies offer, believing in good faith that they are independent experts acting in the interests of education and health.[79]

And the gold threaded seams are luxurious compared to the simple stitching of academic dress. Surely they are worthy of the designer brand cape? They may well be, and they may do important work, but the scene is set here for you to ponder the threads that weave our medical system.

Enter stage left Dr. Jane. She's stretched for time and must keep herself well-versed in so many areas of general medical practice. What she learns about conditions and new treatments, are often created by agents of pharmaceutical companies and transmitted by other agents of those companies. In the end, it matters little how honest our cape-wearing thought leaders are, how much ground-breaking work they do, or how much they believe what they say. They are, inevitably and inescapably, part of large-scale, commercially driven efforts to shape the medical knowledge that physicians like Dr. Jane have and apply in practice.[80]

And conflicts of interest exist *regardless* of whether or not a cape-wearing influencer or pillar of medical society or institution is *actually influenced* by the secondary interest. To disclose such conflicts is a standard industry and ethical practice, but how is a lay person meant to assess research studies in light of declared conflicts of interest of authors?

In fact, transparently declared conflicts could give rise to a perception that research *has been influenced* by third party interests. It's a contentious part of the play and a fine line our experts must tread. But we must shine the spotlight on the subject and remain aware, for it could impact important future research and so have a knock-on effect to our individual healthcare needs.

Our medical societies take their responsibilities seriously and are careful to set out codes of conduct in order to maintain their independence from industry support.[81] But despite such guidelines, ethical dilemmas will appear. According to an article in the British Medical Journal, financial conflicts of interest have repeatedly eroded the credibility of both the medical profession and journals.[82]

Pharmaceutical companies are often cast as the big bad wolf, for good reason as they wield great power, but they also have a valuable role to play. As a woman with a chronic disease, I need big pharma in all their wolf-costume greed and drama. But they should try not to hog the spotlight (or howl at the moon of market supremacy). There's plenty of room on the stage for all players.

"I value the role that pharmaceuticals play in the industry and the FDA," says Dr. Angela DeRosa. "But I wish they wouldn't try to dominate the market, because compounding plays a big role." Despite having her own conflict of interest in this statement as a medical director with Belmar (a large compounding pharmacy) and one she clearly pointed out to me, along with work in her own Hormonal Health Institute, she says, "I wanted to give full disclosure especially as I'm a huge fan of compounding for women when commercial treatments don't meet our unique needs. We should be using medications more appropriately. But we need to look deeper, we need to get the root causes of what's driving it, because a large majority of things that happen as we age are due to hormone deficiencies, we don't need tons of medications, we need hormones."Then, she believes, when hormones are replaced and other things start to happen, we turn to the medications, and they shouldn't be the same.

Different and complementary. And there ends my cautionary tale of how bias and conflict of interest can play out.

6. Not Just Vital for Boy Bands – Testosterone

Like oestrogen and progesterone, testosterone also declines as women age, but it begins to disappear long before perimenopause. A woman in her 40s has on average only half the testosterone circulating in her bloodstream as she does in her 20s.[83] Women start to exhibit symptoms of testosterone deficiency in their 30s, way before the oestrogen deficiency kicks in through their 40s.[84]

So testosterone is essential for a woman's physical and mental wellbeing. It affects ovarian function, bone strength, sexual behaviour including libido, and brain function including mood, sex drive and possibly cognitive function.

I started to wonder why it wasn't an integral part of HRT in perimenopausal women. Surely we must take the loss of testosterone into consideration when treating menopausal symptoms? At this point in my research, the subject seemed like a closed shop. Any reporting on testosterone in women seemed focused on the symptom of low sexual desire or hypoactive sexual desire disorder (HSDD) in postmenopausal women, not for other perimenopausal symptoms. HSDD may not only cause distress, but can have negative effects on personal relationships, quality of life, and general health status.[85]

I didn't understand why the reporting was so centred on this and became quite angry at the lack of information out there. As distressing as

HSDD must be, surely there was more to report from low testosterone levels? This hormone is vital. Sharp knives were avoided.

Looking beyond the headline symptoms of decreased libido and sexual responsiveness, I found reports that testosterone-deficient pre- and postmenopausal women may also experience a range of other symptoms including anxiety, irritability, depression, unexplained fatigue, lack of wellbeing, changes in cognition and memory loss. Plus insomnia, hot flashes, rheumatoid complaints, pain, vaginal dryness, urinary complaints and incontinence.[86]

I scratched a little deeper and found snippets of positive information on the benefits of testosterone therapy, breadcrumbs that led me to consult a doctor who specialised in women's health and menopause. She had also been through menopause. I took full blood screen results with me.

After a thorough consultation and reviewing my recent blood test results, she prescribed an iron supplement to boost iron stores, which were within range but on the low end. She also changed my synthetic progesterone tablet to the bioidentical or 'body-identical' micronised progesterone soft capsule called Prometrium – an exact duplicate of human progesterone, as it has fewer side effects (as already discussed).

This doctor also gave me an *off-label* prescription (see below) for a female testosterone cream called AndroFeme® 1 per cent. She had used testosterone with other peri- and postmenopausal patients; some found tremendous relief from brain fog, fatigue and low-libido and some saw little or no improvement. It required blood tests every few weeks to check levels, along with breast screening and a PAP smear. At this point I was desperate for energy and brain function, so it had to be worth a shot.

Seven to ten days into testosterone therapy, the fog started to clear and I began to feel far less fatigued. Since commencing treatment my life has turned around, I have more vitality and mental clarity. I'm no longer despairing of my inability to function as a normal human being, and I've regained my sense of self. I lost so much confidence with my cognitive slide, and the physical fatigue made me feel like a train wreck. It was one of the lowest (and most confusing) points of my life.

One size does not fit all

I came off it for a week after an abnormally high blood test, while we retested.[87] My memory started to slip again and my energy depleted, despite the additional iron supplement. I felt the slide back to horrible begin. A smaller dose was administered.

The high results appeared again in between other normal to low results, which was confusing and worrying, so my doctor referred me to Associate Professor John Eden, who is a gynaecologist and reproductive endocrinologist (meaning he specialises in women's hormones).

I feel like my old self when I'm using it, so I really wanted to get this therapy right. Professor Eden felt that the results may have been incorrect or due to the fact I was using the cream on my inner arms, the site of the blood sample collection. I've since learned that there is much contention between medical professionals over testing levels and interpretation of those.

Some suggest that routinely monitoring testosterone levels and adjusting therapy based on a single value should be viewed with scepticism. And that dosing should be based on clinical efficacy, similar to insulin dosing, where individual biologic effect and tolerability determines the dose rather than testing blood serum levels.[88] As a woman with type 1 diabetes, I can agree with that! My insulin requirements and blood sugar levels vary according to many different factors on any given day. The results constantly change.

And this is what's so confusing about differing opinions in the medical profession over hormone deficiency, thyroid, perimenopause, what works and what doesn't. Hormones are very complex, and what works for one may have no effect or be dangerous in another. That's why I'm sharing this information with you, so you can ask questions of your healthcare practitioners. And to see that there are many differing opinions and no one definitive answer.

For example, my menopause specialist warned that an excess of testosterone can have a permanent effect of a deeper voice, male pattern baldness, acne and also cause excess body hair. In fact these side effects are mentioned often in press articles, academic papers and by menopause societies and doctors, but other medical professionals disagree. Some research has shown that in a trial of women patients on testosterone implant therapy for more than a year, it had no effect on the female voice, a mild increase in facial hair and only a minor increase in acne. Interestingly, 50 percent of patients reported moister, softer skin and fewer wrinkles.[89] Sounds like a skincare ad. I know, I'm rolling my eyes.

I still have a full head of hair, female dulcet tones and haven't suffered any noticeable side effects. But I've been using it for less than a year. Some professionals say; 'we don't know the long-term effects' and some say; 'we've been using it successfully for the past 80 years without major issues.'

I had a few teenage zits at the very start, but that's not unusual for me (it's so unfair when you're 50!) and I also had very sore, sensitive breasts for a week or so, but that was all. No extra facial fur happening here, just the usual odd and annoying stray mid-life whisker sprouting out of nowhere.

A medical maze

You need to ask questions of your medical practitioners and advocate for your own wellbeing. Too many women are dismissed by doctors who aren't well-versed in perimenopause or menopause, you must get prepared to find your way through the maze.

Professor Eden is adamant that we need to normalise the discussion and treatment of menopausal women because without treatment, too many women will suffer ongoing hot flashes and other debilitating symptoms.

During our mid-afternoon telehealth consultation, he admitted the majority of the women he had seen that day were being slammed by their symptoms. When he said his tissue box is regularly emptied by patients, I fully empathised with them, because that had been me, weeping and desperate, back in 2019 before beginning treatment.

HRT and testosterone combined has helped me to feel so much like my old self again. And despite the fact that some clinicians and medical societies continue to report that there's not enough evidence to support the use of testosterone therapy in women for anything other than sexual dysfunction, I have the energy to walk up stairs now, plus go for 16-kilometre bike rides and take brisk walks with our dog.

I'm still lazy (I don't think there's a drug for that?) and I have to push myself to get off my perimenopausal lardy arse. I'm not fanging around like a 18-year-old lad! (I've got one of those and he's got way more energy and testosterone than his mother, and quite rightly so.)

My brain function has not fully returned yet, but at ten months into testosterone therapy treatment it's 80 per cent back to pre-peri, which is an enormous improvement. Enormous. I feel human again even if I'm not razor-sharp; I can still be slow to get my head around concepts and respond with clarity to in-depth discussion or debate. That's my excuse, and I'm sticking to it.

Off-label prescriptions

I also spoke with Michael Buckley, a pharmacist and the medical director of Lawley Pharmaceuticals in Western Australia, who has worked for years towards TGA approval of a female testosterone product. Their male product was approved in 2015. As this book goes to press in late November 2020, AndroFeme® 1 per cent has just received approval to be included on the Australian Register of Therapeutic Goods (ARTG) for the management of HSDD in postmenopausal women.

It's the first approval of its kind in the world and a big deal, as the medical profession are now freer to prescribe testosterone for women, and by April 2021 it's expected to be available nationally from all Australian pharmacies. Hopefully other governing regulatory bodies for drugs across the world will follow suit with approval, even if that approval is only recommended to treat HSDD. It's a step in the right direction.

Those who want it for anything other than HSDD, like me, will need to find a doctor who is prepared to prescribe it 'off-label'. And of course, it may not be the right therapy for you.

Testosterone by prescription

Until recently a female-specific testosterone product hadn't been approved by any regulatory authority in the world, making it very difficult to convince doctors to write a prescription despite the evidence (discussed earlier in the chapter). But due to legislative differences between Western Australia (WA) and the Commonwealth of Australia, AndroFeme® 1 per cent was exempted from inclusion on the Australian Register of Therapeutic Goods (ARTG) and could therefore be dispensed in WA.

Lawley Pharmaceuticals has been licenced to manufacture and supply this product to pharmacies in WA since 1999. I'm in New South Wales (NSW) and I currently have my prescription dispensed direct from the manufacturer by mail from WA.

On the 20th November 2020, Lawley Pharmaceuticals obtained approval by the Therapeutic Goods Administration (TGA) for registration of AndroFeme® 1 per cent in the ARTG, for use in Australia with postmenopausal women who suffer HSDD.

For women with other symptoms it can be prescribed off-label, which means for a use that doesn't have specific approval by the TGA. The TGA advise doctors to use caution when considering prescribing medicines for anything other than the use it's approved for. This means the individual doctor carries the risks involved with prescribing off-label and so they will often refer you to a specialist for advice and prescriptions. See Chapter 9 for more information on finding the right doctor to help you. AndroFeme® 1 per cent is expected to be available throughout Australia from April 2020.

Unfortunately, without peer-reviewed scientific evidence from clinical trials (usually funded by big pharmaceutical companies), it's unlikely that any regulatory body will approve a testosterone product for use in *pre- or perimenopausal* women, despite data up to five years that shows no adverse effect in healthy women after menopause.[90]

Ok, so we understand there's one commercial testosterone product available for women in Australia via WA and nationally in April 2021, which doctors can prescribe for HSDD or 'off-label' for anything else and that carries risk, so most don't. Let's have a look at why this is the case.

The plot thickens

In September 2019, the Endocrine Society published in their *Journal of Clinical Endocrinology & Metabolism* (JCEM) a Global Consensus Position Statement on the use of testosterone treatment in women. The panel of medical professionals concluded that evidence exists for beneficial effects of testosterone therapy in postmenopausal women only, specifically those suffering with hypoactive sexual desire disorder (HSDD). Hence why the topic of HSDD appeared when I began to research the use of testosterone in women.

The panel also highlighted the pressing need for more research into testosterone therapy for women and the development and licensing of products indicated specifically for women.[91] Amen to that. But they also concluded that, at present, the available evidence does not support the use of testosterone for the treatment of any symptom or medical condition other than HSDD.

This is interesting because the data presented included selected *industry-sponsored* randomised controlled trials (RCTs) but excluded other research such as observational studies. Reconciling the results between the two is a challenge for clinical medicine and is important in this discussion. RCTs collect data under ideal conditions among a highly selected and qualified group, but observational studies tend to measure the effects of a treatment in 'real world' settings.[92] Both offer useful data, but sometimes the results differ.

Observational studies are particularly valuable for clinical situations unlikely to be tested using RCTs, and many provide valid evidence, although RCT's are considered to be the gold standard by researchers as a more reliable way to collect and interpret the data. Both types of research have their place in evaluating therapeutic outcomes and in fact a recent Cochrane review[93] found little evidence that the results of observational studies and RCTs systematically disagreed.

The committee's recommendations after reviewing selected RCT's (and excluding certain data from observational studies) advised against compounded therapies, dosing, subcutaneous testosterone implants, and injections although no supporting data nor 'evidence of harm' was presented.

Other medical professionals criticise the authors of this review for not including observational studies or case reports, and for not acknowledging the theoretical and observed benefits of testosterone in the prevention and treatment of breast cancer.[94] The use of testosterone to help women with anything other than HSDD is controversial despite it being prescribed for more than 80 years.[95]

Professor Susan Davis, endocrinologist and president of the International Menopause Society, was a leading author of the consensus statement. She has made an important contribution to the understanding of the role of androgens and oestrogens in multiple non-reproductive target tissues. I shared an early draft of this book with her prior to release, and she was vocal about misinformation around menopause in the media. This caused me to delay publishing and re-check my research and information. Plus, my personal experience didn't tally up with the recommendations of the panel, I wanted to report what I learned about that and why it can be so difficult to access the right treatment for our individual menopausal symptoms.

Dr. Davis also led researchers to create a systematic review of data collected from 46 reports on 36 trials of testosterone involving 8,480 women, to look at benefits and risks of testosterone therapy for women. The results were published in 2019 and showed that postmenopausal women who experience a reduction in sexual desire that causes them personal concern or distress may benefit from testosterone therapy.

In regard to the effects of testosterone on wellbeing, mood and cognition in postmenopausal women, the review concluded that there is insufficient evidence to support the use of testosterone to enhance cognitive performance or to delay cognitive decline. It also stated that the effects of testosterone on individual wellbeing and musculoskeletal and cognitive health, as well as long-term safety, warrant further investigation.[96] I believe this is vital.

In premenopausal women the review also reported that testosterone may improve wellbeing, but the data was inconclusive. It said data did not show an effect of testosterone on depressed mood. However it is the case that many clinicians (in real world settings) report seeing positive results on testosterone and depression.[97]

"It's maddening to me that we continue to sedate women with antidepressants when we need to treat the underlying cause, which is hormone deficiency," says Dr. DeRosa. And that although some women can't go on oestrogen, for reasons of breast cancer or other indications, there are very rare limitations to use testosterone, which can help with a lot of menopausal symptoms. She believes it would be far better for them than using an antidepressant.

Regardless of the differences of opinion that I discovered while researching this book, most seem to agree that there is a need for an approved testosterone product for women. Professor Davis believes the beneficial effects for postmenopausal women's sex lives and personal wellbeing underlines the validity of this.[98] "There is irrefutable evidence that testosterone therapy, at a dose that results in premenopausal blood testosterone levels in postmenopausal women, can be highly effective for the treatment of postmenopausal women with low sexual desire and associated personal distress, or HSDD," Professor Davis said.[99]

A range of products to suit individual women's needs and available across the world would be ideal. Compounded or commercial, patches, creams, pellets, whatever works to help us. I'm using AndroFeme® 1 per cent cream as a delivery system, it isn't perfect as it spikes on application and declines throughout the day, so I'm currently splitting the dose into two, applying it at the start and end of my day. However I'm very grateful that I can access this product. Testosterone pellets inserted under the skin are another option that have both advantages and disadvantages – I plan to explore those – stay tuned via my Facebook group*.

Clearly there is an urgent need to address all the available evidence for using testosterone to treat anything other than HSDD in women. Perhaps it would have more exploration demanded if men suffered through menopause.

If you are suffering from a loss of sexual desire, have dryness, discomfort or pain during sex, are less responsive to sexual stimulation and find this distressing, then it's worth seeking treatment. It's more than just sex; it impacts wellbeing too. If you're postmenopausal or haven't had a period for 12 months, then you may be eligible to try testosterone therapy for HSDD; speak with your doctor or check out this fact sheet**.

I don't have the definitive low-down on how menopause is going to play out for me. So I'm doing my due diligence and checking out the natural and lifestyle options I can use to support me as I continue through postmenopause. I may not stay on hormone therapy in the long term but for now, I like that I'm no longer utterly debilitated by symptoms, and that hormone therapy protects my heart and bone density. I'm also a nicer human, mostly. Plus I've heaps more energy, and it's rare that I suffer hot flashes or night sweats.

Okay, so next up, let's take a look at non-hormone therapy options.

*https://www.facebook.com/groups/secretmensesbusiness
**https://www.menopause.org.au/health-info/resources/1484-testosterone-and-women

7. Alternatives to Hormone Therapies

If you can't or don't want to use HRT, then you may wish to explore non-hormone medications or complementary/herbal therapies to help you to manage the symptoms. These alternatives may help some women and not others, but everything is worth looking at if perimenopause is turning you into someone you don't recognise reflected back in the mirror, a blithering, damp puddle of your former glory.

Or, if you aren't yet experiencing symptoms, then consider what might help build some resilience to support your endocrine system. Care should be taken as therapies can interact with current conditions and treatments, and even though some derive from natural sources, even those may have side effects. Seek professional advice before making your decision on treatment.

Non-hormone prescription medications

If you have severe symptoms and cannot use HRT for medical reasons, the Australasian Menopause Society (AMS) suggests discussing these alternatives with your doctor. Remember my note in the interlude that conflicts of interest exist regardless of whether or not any medical society or institute is actually influenced by the secondary interest, no matter the intent. I'm not suggesting any medical societies nor individual medical professionals are biased, but that you are mindful of any declared conflicts of interest. If they concern you in regard to treatment then discuss them with your doctor.

Antidepressants

A low dose of some types of antidepressant have been used for many years, helping around 70 per cent of women to reduce severe hot flashes and night sweats.[100] Again, Dr. DeRosa believes that we should be treating the underlying cause of hormone deficiency and using testosterone when oestrogen is not appropriate. Be sure to ask about side effects, and make sure you're not being fobbed off with antidepressants because you appear to be depressed by symptoms. It's normal to have emotional mood swings when your hormones are all kinds of crazy. But take your doctor's advice if you are depressed.[101]

> ### *Consider this:*
>
> Dr. DeRosa believes using high blood pressure meds, epilepsy treatments or antihistamines is medically reckless, as many are significant medications with tremendous risks and side effects. "When oestrogen can't be safely used, testosterone alone can alleviate a large majority of the menopausal symptoms, even the ones that are primarily caused by estrogen loss. It will lessen hot flashes and it may not get rid of them, but they are usually markedly improved. It won't really help with vaginal dryness, but vaginal estrogen can be used to help with this."

High blood pressure meds

Clonidine is a medication that has been used for nearly 50 years and can help those with high blood pressure, ADHD and anxiety. This medication can help some women with mild menopausal symptoms. Other than hormonal preparations, only Clonidine has been TGA approved for treatment of hot flashes.[102] Consider the risks and side effects of using this.

Epilepsy treatments

Epilepsy drugs (gabapentin and pregabalin) have been used for many years to treat epilepsy and nerve pain and are reported to have few side effects. These medications have shown a mild to moderate effect on reducing hot flashes in women with a history of breast cancer.[103] Consider the risks and side effects of using these drugs.

Emerging treatments

This AMS fact sheet* outlines a few emerging treatments: one involving antihistamines.[104] Small studies have shown that a widely available antihistamine (cetirizine) might help some women with menopausal symptoms. At this stage, more research is needed to confirm this as a future treatment option and note, Dr. DeRosa says that these medications are not without side-effects such as sedation, vaginal dryness and blunted orgasm.

Melatonin

Melatonin is a hormone that helps strengthen and improve sleep-wake cycles, making it easier to sleep on a regular schedule. Peri- and postmenopausal women often complain of insomnia, which is presumed due to decreased levels of estrogen, and possibly melatonin.[105] Healthy sleep maintenance supports other processes that happen during your sleep and aids liver function.[106] In Australia you need a prescription, but you can buy it over the counter in many other countries (in liquid and tablet form). I've used melatonin to help with jet-lag after long-haul

*https://www.menopause.org.au/health-info/fact-sheets/non-hormonal-treatment-options-for-menopausal-symptoms

trips and have recently started using it at bedtime. My sleep is much improved.

Herbal therapies

Various herbal remedies have been found to help some women, although many are not supported by *formal evidence* as expensive clinical trials have not been undertaken. You may find some that work for you. Be careful to check with your doctor that any supplements won't interact with your prescribed medications.

My doctor says complementary and herbal therapies are a grey area in general medicine; he's seen good outcomes for some patients who can't get results from or take prescription medications to relieve symptoms. If you are using herbal or botanic therapies, do your own research; you can search for clinical trial results at the Cochrane Library*. The AMS website** contains some useful information. You will find more detail on the following:

Black cohosh

This perennial plant native to North America has a long history of use. Native Americans used it to treat various ailments including menstrual irregularities[107] and European settlers used it as a tonic to support women's reproductive health.[108] But there are varying reports of its efficacy of treating menopausal symptoms.[109]

In 2007, the Australian Department of Health began requiring that products containing black cohosh carry a warning that this ingredient may harm the liver in some individuals.[110]

---

*https://www.cochranelibrary.com/
**https://www.menopause.org.au/hp/information-sheets/734-complementary-and-herbal-therapies-for-hot-flushes

Phytoestrogens including red clover

Short-term studies suggest benefit in using phytoestrogens (plant oestrogens) including red clover early in menopause, but good long-term studies are lacking. They may interfere with treatments for breast cancer.[111]

Wild yam cream, evening primrose oil, flaxseed and ginseng

Very limited data exists on the use of wild yam cream, evening primrose oil, flaxseed and ginseng for hot flashes. Ginseng can reduce the effects of immunosuppressive and other drugs.[112]

Maca root

I've heard perimenopausal women report that maca root is a useful supplement for cognitive function. According to the AMS poor quality trials indicate improvement in menopausal symptom scores, but there's no sufficient evidence to support the use of maca.[113] However I found a trial that showed Maca JDS, a proprietary maca blend, doubles the effect on cognitive function compared to placebo. The trial states that it can provide a safe way to improve cognitive function, offering overall enhanced executive functioning, which is important for focus, organisation, memory, and flexible thinking.[114] Hell yeah, don't we all need that! I am planning to try this option soon, I'll keep you posted via Facebook*.

Pine bark, pollen extract and Siberian rhubarb

Some women use pine bark, pollen extract and Siberian rhubarb to relieve symptoms, and further research is needed to establish efficacy and safety.[115] Proceed at your own risk.

*https://www.facebook.com/groups/secretmensesbusiness

St John's wort

St John's wort is a perennial herb that has been used to treat nervous conditions since ancient Greek times. I found a small study of 70 women showing that it reduced hot flashes, menopausal symptoms, and depression in postmenopausal women.[116] The AMS states that St John's wort can be effective for depression, but it may also interact with other medicines, so always seek medical advice before using.[117]

Essential oils

Some plant-based essential oils contain phytoestrogens that behave in a similar way to oestrogen. Women have used them to relieve symptoms although evidential support does not yet exist.[118]

Non-herbal therapies

Non-herbal remedies include:

- zinc
- vitamin E
- omega-3
- magnesium
- homeopathy.

The AMS states that non-herbal therapies do not relieve menopausal symptoms according to the evidence, but some people claim to experience benefits when using them.[119] I take a bunch of vitamins including magnesium, zinc, vitamins C, D, and B and a liquid iron supplement. I generally feel better when I take them and a bit smug every time I pee and see the bright yellow stream of vitamins. Some say that's very expensive urine.

Complementary therapies

Conventional medicine tends to take a 'reactive' approach to treat symptoms when they hit, so it's unlikely you would consult a doctor when feeling well. But why not take a 'proactive' approach? This is what the Brownie mantra is all about. Remember our motto 'Be prepared?'

Complementary therapies – naturopathy, chiropractic, massage, homeopathy, etc. – may be used in conjunction with conventional medications. The AMS reports that certain complementary and herbal therapies may have benefits, while others have shown no effect.

I'm a great believer in trying therapies that appeal to you when you need help. They can offer positive benefits to your mind, body and spirit. Use common sense and ask for recommendations and qualified practitioners.

Limited evidence suggests that hypnosis might improve menopausal symptoms, but no evidence exists that acupuncture, magnetic therapy, reflexology or chiropractic interventions are effective.[120] That doesn't mean you won't find a therapy that works well for you.

Example: A naturopathic approach

Whatever treatment – medication, herb, vitamin or supplement – you decide to use, make sure you do it with the guidance of a qualified professional, keeping in mind your situation, medical history and background. Here's an example of the approach a naturopath might take to your wellbeing. Naturopaths tend to take a proactive approach and may first look at stressors in a mid-life female patient's life that might be unbalancing the endocrine system.[121]

Our adrenal glands are part of the endocrine system, and they become the prime producers of oestrogen and progesterone during the transitional years to menopause, when our ovaries stop working. They also produce other vital hormones including cortisol, the fight or flight stress hormone.

So our adrenals need to be in optimum shape for the work required. Many of us are working full time, raising children and juggling myriad demands in our daily lives. Stressed-out adrenals compromise their function to secrete oestrogens, androgens and other vital hormones. I wish I had understood this sooner!

Are your adrenals fighting fit, or are they battling and a bit knackered?

Mine were definitely overworked and underpaid. Hormones are easily unbalanced by poor sleep patterns, food and lifestyle choices,[122] so a naturopath will look at ways to rebalance, alongside liver and gut health – both of which metabolise our hormones. They might order more blood tests, alongside the usual full blood screens required by doctors. From here they will look to herbal medicine, vitamins, minerals and other complementary therapies to support the whole body in navigating your hormonal transition.

Your body, your choice

So in summary, options other than hormones are available to explore, but what works for some may not necessarily work for others. Preventative or proactive measures are definitely a great option to give yourself the best chance for resilience and a better experience through perimenopause. If they don't work, you can also consider medical options outside usual hormone therapy.

Personally, after a period of crash-and-burn in my mid-40s, I began a proactive, holistic approach to my health, knowing it would help with aging. I consulted a naturopath, a homeopath and a therapist to work through challenges. I restarted my old exercise regime and made cleaner health choices to support myself in staying well. But stress, workload and life poured down like a violent storm, overwhelming me and washing away all of those good pathways I'd created. I dropped the ball on my self-care at a crucial time just prior to perimenopause. This was a huge mistake.

It forced me into a reactive corner, where I took the medical path as a last resort. Without HRT *and* testosterone to deal with my symptoms I would have ended up in that straightjacket for sure. The million-dollar question is, would I have suffered such devastating symptoms if I had been at the top of my wellbeing game? I don't know, but I am certain I would have had more resilience to cope with the changes rather than beginning from a place of utter depletion.

Next up, we continue this theme of preserving our health and wellbeing. Let's treat our bodies like the temples they are, giving them thanks for their amazing abilities. There's an etiquette for visiting a temple, and it involves respecting the sacred place of worship. Are you respecting yours?

8. Your Body Is a Temple

Your body has seen you through some adventures, and you've probably abused it through your life at times. Maybe you eat clean, run marathons and drink copious amounts of water and green tea. If you're anything like me, though, you're probably partial to coffee, wine, and Cheezos, and run only in extreme circumstances, like out of the front door to the car when you're late.

A bit of indulgence is ok, in limited amounts. These bodies we inhabit are amazing things, but they can only suffer so much abuse before failing us. And we need them functioning better than ever through perimenopause and into old age. I wish I had entered perimenopause as fit and well-functioning as I was at age 40.

If you're in your 40s, take the challenge to get fit and healthy now! And if you're in peri- or postmenopause, do it anyway. It's never too late to haul a lardy arse upright and shake your booty. By improving your resilience, you may better tolerate symptoms. Less stabbing, road rage and mid-life alcoholics in the community has to be a win-win.

Exercise and maintain healthy weight

Evidence suggests that weight gain increases the severity of vasomotor symptoms (hot flashes, night sweats), so *maintaining a healthy weight might be helpful*. Easily said. Right now, I just need to look at carbs to gain more pounds. Pass me a celery stick with that Prosecco. Is that dust gathering on my treadmill?

Exercising relieves stress and helps build fitness and muscle mass, which burns more energy (even when snoring!) And it staves off additional weight gain, which is also good for bone health. It's hard to be motivated when you're feeling exhausted, but regular physical activity can help make symptoms more manageable and regain some control.

Pelvic floor exercises (Kegels) will also help with those leaky sneezes,[123] or for better results, a physical therapist can help train you to contract and release the right muscles for a supple and functional pelvic floor. Other benefits to exercise include the following:

- Strength training from weights at the gym or dumbbells and resistance tubing at home will boost your metabolism and build bone and muscle strength. Dinner lady arms, lookout![124]
- Cardio will help raise your heart rate to improve heart and lung health and burn calories and fat. Take regular brisk walks, cycle, swim, jog, dance to '70s disco or just run up and down on the spot.[125]
- Yoga helps you to stay cool, calm and collected, and it helps keep your nervous system balanced. Plus you can maintain strength without overheating into flash dance mode! So, for obvious reasons, you should avoid the hot room Bikram-style yoga![126] The combination of relaxation, meditation and exercise helps some women, particularly with mood swings because it relieves stress, which tends to make emotions and flashes run hot.

And who wouldn't benefit by stretching their aching muscles? Being able to touch your toes easily must be comforting and soothing. I don't know about that. But I know I should start yoga again so I can be smug about my flexibility when I'm 60 and show off my svelteness on Instagram by wearing sleeveless shirts, and so should you.

Change and clear your mind

The good news is that evidence shows cognitive behaviour therapy (CBT) improves wellbeing and decreases the impact of menopausal symptoms.[127] CBT can help you change unhelpful ways of thinking, feeling and behaving. According to the Australasian Menopause Society (AMS), studies suggest that CBT can help you cope with the impact of menopausal symptoms while also increasing your wellbeing. Look to CBT groups or professional psychotherapists[128] for this sort of therapy.

> ### *Three steps to stress relief*
>
> Emotional wellbeing is essential in decreasing stress levels, as is exercise, healthy eating and sleep patterns.
>
> 1. Recognise what your stressors are: external factors (work, relationships, environment), nutritional, lifestyle and emotional.
> 2. Identify ways you can manage those stressors. Make a list.
> 3. Begin to take those actions. By managing stress, you can alleviate the impact on your internal physical systems, glands, organs etc.

Meditation helps me through many challenges in life because I pile expectations on myself and sink into the quicksand of overwhelm. I seemed to suffer anxiety heaps more through perimenopause, and many women say the same thing. Meditation, or mindfulness meditation[129] is so great. And it gives me the excuse of some quiet 'me-time'. I highly recommend noise cancelling headphones to tune out the world around you.

Checkout my Facebook page* for links to playlists and you'll find more about that and many other ideas for transforming your life in my book, *The Naked Truth About YOU***.

*https://www.facebook.com/susannemitchellauthor/
**http://www.susanne-mitchell.com/

Prioritise sleep

If you sleep well, your liver can more easily process things at night, and you'll get great flow through as your organs have a chance to do their job unhindered. Going to bed at the same time every night and getting up at the same time every morning is one of the best things you can do for your adrenal system and your general wellbeing.[130] Minimise things like coffee, alcohol and screen time at bedtime too. I also take my prescribed Prometrium, Estrogel and also a melatonin tablet at bedtime and my sleep is much improved.

Make better food choices

You might rely on food for comfort, then the depleted energy levels turn exercise into a marathon effort. It can be a vicious circle. Make better food choices by including protein, omega-3 fatty acids, fibre, and calcium in your diet. Limit saturated fats, highly refined carbs, and sugar. Try to avoid packaged and processed foods, and drink more water. Cut down caffeine, alcohol and spicy foods, which are known to trigger sweating and hot flashes.

Nigel Denby is an award-winning dietician, with special clinical interests in menopause and women's hormonal health, if you want to find ways to eat better, take a look here*.

Fasting is a mighty good way for your body to recover from the constant processing through your gut. A healthy sleep regime is a form of fasting which can easily be extended by drinking only water or herbal tea for the first few hours of the day. But please don't follow random fasting plans you find on the internet or in women's magazines (some can be dangerous). Dr Michael Mosley has done some great work in

*https://www.nigeldenbydietitian.co.uk/

this area; check out his book and website*. **Make sure you consult your doctor if you're planning to fast.**

Restrict alcohol intake

Many of us turn to alcohol to soften the despair and mood swings. Nice women in menopause support groups on Facebook agree that to lessen symptoms it helps to stop drinking. WHAT DO THEY MEAN, STOP DRINKING?

We are the nation (Australia) that kept bottle shops open during lockdown as an essential service. But apparently it helps to stop leaning on the booze. We should have stabbing booths filled with fake, straw-filled partners as part of our rehab. I mean seriously. We could piggyback them with a mobile breast screening service. Get your breasts checked and vent your perimenopausal anger to keep your loved ones safe.

But seriously, so many women are terrified of taking HRT when the risk of breast cancer is less than in those who have that second glass of wine or are over a healthy weight range and are sloth-like in their exercise regime.

I am making a conscious effort to change my behaviour despite the disadvantage that my default spirit animal is a sloth slash hedgehog. Lazy and prickly at times.

Tonight, I may drink wine with dinner and aim to keep it to one (probably large-ish) glass. There's always room for improvement, but I don't whip myself over everything. But as I age and manage my chronic disease, I try a little harder to behave. The healthier you are the easier any transition will be.

*https://thefast800.com/

Ditch the smokes

If you're a smoker, now is the time to quit. Back when I stopped, I used nicotine vapes to start as an easy replacement of the fags with less chemicals, then graduated to nicotine gum because it gave me that hit instantly *and* helped replace the hand-to-mouth habit of the vapes. Exercise helped, as did the MyQuitBuddy* app that encouraged me along the way. You can make the choice to do it!

Tips for worshipping at the altar of your body

Some simple tips for worship:

- Aim to drink more water than coffee, alcohol, soft drinks or smoothies
- Give up the smokes, vapes or drugs and limit booze
- Make sure you walk or take some form of exercise daily or at least three times a week
- Learn to manage your mental health, meditate, journal, take therapy or do something creative to switch off your noisy thinking mind
- Aim for early nights and healthy sleeping patterns
- Never go food shopping when you're hungry, it's dangerous (last week I bought a huge bag of Cheezos – there's none left)
- Identify small things that nurture you and do them; think, reading, soaking in the bath, throwing custard pies at your gobby kids, walking in nature, moisturising your hair and skin, stretching or yoga.

Start treating your precious body more like a temple to worship rather than a submissive to whip. Your hormones can dominate, but poor lifestyle choices will begin to show (if they haven't already).

*https://www.health.gov.au/resources/apps-and-tools/my-quitbuddy-app

As I write this I'm drinking a coffee because I'm under deadline and a tad stretched stress-wise. But I'll go and grab a glass of water next and plan to get out for a dog walk in the morning before hitting the computer for another day. It's a balance.

I'm conscious of what goes into my body, but I'm not perfect. And I vehemently wish that I'd hit perimenopause in tip-top shape, on top of my game. I didn't, but if you're not in it yet, you can.

9. What to Take to Your Doctor

Menopause is a natural part of a woman's life. It is not a medical issue. If your symptoms are mild and not affecting your daily life, you may not feel the need to consult a doctor. But as you approach or head through midlife, it's worth a maintenance check regardless of symptoms.

A doctor will evaluate your symptoms and any change in the pattern of menstrual bleeding to make a clinical assessment of whether you are perimenopausal or have passed through menopause into postmenopause. Other routine tests and checks may be ordered to rule out other conditions.[131] If your symptoms are impacting on your quality of life, then don't suffer in silence, get yourself seen.

Firstly, what kind of doctor should you see?

Start by finding the official menopause society in your part of the world, they may have funding conflicts, but they also provide some useful information. The International Menopause Society has a list.[132] Some countries have government-funded menopause centres, so check what's available locally for targeted help. Alternatively, look for a doctor specialising in women's health by searching the internet for 'women's health clinic' or 'sexual health clinic'.

The AMS has a list of doctors in Australia who have a special interest in women's health in midlife and menopause, and the promotion of healthy aging. If you're in the USA, you can search for healthcare professionals who specialise through perimenopause and beyond on the North American Menopause Society (NAMS) website.

The British Menopause Society (BMS) has launched a UK-wide register of BMS recognised menopause specialists*, covering both NHS and private clinics and services. Note that the BMS has a disclaimer stating it does not endorse compounded bioidentical treatments on its 'find-a-menopause-specialist' page. Remember that you have the power to question and make your own informed decisions with regard to your healthcare.

Or you can go to your family doctor. I regularly hear stories from women about how there is a chronic lack of understanding of perimenopause in general medical practice. So make sure you're educated on the subject before making your appointment, and who knows? You may get lucky and find some great help via your local clinic.

Some doctors are brilliant and some less so. They have short windows of time for patients and often heavy workloads. But this is no excuse for bad service. You have the same worth as someone going through puberty, cancer, chronic pain, childbirth, injury or the next person in the waiting room. Stand tall, perimenopausal warrior women, but leave your sword at home for all our sakes.

My male doctor attended a women's health conference soon after I melted in a puddle in his surgery, because he said he clearly needed to become more informed about new treatments in perimenopause. Now that's a great outcome!

Be prepared

I'm so far beyond my Girl Scout years, but this motto continues to serve. It's best to be prepared before turning up regardless of who you

*https://thebms.org.uk/find-a-menopause-specialist/

go and see. Consider the outcome you want before going in; how are you feeling, do you need some kind of intervention? Are you hoping to walk away with a script for HRT? Or do you want a referral to a doctor specialising in women's health and menopause? Or to find a doctor who is open to prescribing testosterone or (if you aren't in Australia) will prescribe compounded bioidentical hormone therapy? I've often called ahead to ask similar questions prior to booking in.

Take a list of symptoms, mild, moderate or horrible, and note how they are affecting your work, family life and relationships. Night sweats, vaginal dryness, aching joints, loss of libido, itchy skin or vag, worse-than-normal PMS, hot flashes, weak pelvic floor or poor brain function? Are they triggered by anything, or does a particular situation make them better or worse?

By the time I went to see a specialist menopause doctor, I had written a rough timeline of what had happened when and gave it to the doctor to read before we went through everything. A lot had happened as I had been in perimenopause for a few years by then. It meant she was well informed of the overview and timing before looking at specifics. My brain was misfiring with fog and so the list meant I didn't forget anything.

Check this list of menopause symptoms* to see if any apply to you, and educate yourself further with other fact sheets** from the Australasian Menopause Society.

Ask for a full health check and blood work as this will provide a range of information about your overall health and is a smart idea at mid-life anyway. Make sure they include thyroid (TSH, T4 and ask for T3 too, it's not on Medicare in Australia) as thyroid hormones can mimic menopausal symptoms. Your doctor may not test for hormone levels if you are older than 45 or haven't had a period for a year as they

* https://www.menopause.org.au/health-info/fact-sheets/menopause-what-are-the-symptoms
**https://www.menopause.org.au/hp/information-sheets

are clinical indicators of menopause; anyway, levels can fluctuate and are unlikely to change their management.

Perimenopause and antidepressants

Perimenopause can be written off as the patient just being depressed due to mood swings, and antidepressants may then be prescribed. If this happens and you a) aren't trying to find a non-hormone drug to treat hot flashes and b) don't feel depressed, yet are frustrated and feeling low with symptoms, then ask why they are suggesting antidepressants. You are allowed to question. It's healthy to look out for yourself. There may be good reason for the suggestion, so if you are depressed then consider your doctor's advice.

So once you've read up and educated yourself on perimenopause, make your appointment. It's worth scheduling a double-length appointment so you have enough time to go through everything.

Consider asking your partner or a friend to come along to support and to prompt you, it's easy to forget when you're feeling anxious. I've also heard some women report they had a more sympathetic response when a partner was able to talk about the effect their perimenopause was having on him/her/they.

Here's the checklist of things to take:

1. A list of symptoms and how they are affecting you.
2. A timeline of any changes in your period, cycle and symptoms occurring.
3. A list of questions you have around perimenopause. This might include lifestyle, diet, exercise or medication.
4. A list of embarrassing questions you might have about intimate

matters like sex, intercourse, libido. They've heard it all, so don't let embarrassment hinder your treatment. You could write these down and hand them a note if it's hard to say out loud or in front of your appointment buddy.

5. A list of questions or concerns you may have about different treatments and medications.

6. A list of any other medications or natural therapies that you are currently taking.

Perimenopause can have a huge impact on you physically, mentally and emotionally. It can affect your home and work lives, so be sure to share all aspects with your doctor. If there's anything you don't understand, don't be afraid to ask them to repeat or explain further.

Next up, you might be surprised to learn that changes associated with aging and menopause vary both historically and across cultures. Let's consider how we can help our (Western) society to adapt the way menopause is perceived, understood and managed.

10. Let's Embrace the Renewal Years

In Western societies, we generally view menopause as the end of our youthful bloom. We dry up, get narky and become advertising targets for incontinence knickers and funeral insurance. And we are raised to buy into the idea that aging is an undesirable destination, the wrong side of town, you don't want to venture *there*. You might get stabbed by an angry perimenopausal woman trying to cope with that indefinable thing they've lost. Now where the hell did I leave my (youthful) feminine power this time?

No wonder we struggle to admit what we're going through. The idea of becoming an aging creature past your sell-by date with cobwebs across your V-jay is confronting. But it doesn't have to be this way. Let's break this tired old stereotype of post-menopausal life.

The Japanese word for the menopause life phase is *konenki*, which translates to renewal years and energy. One study found Mayan women, although they experience uncomfortable symptoms, look forward to menopause, as it provides newfound freedom and status.[133] Indeed in many cultures, menopause is seen as a time of new respect and freedom for women.

Why don't we, in Western society, adopt this view? If we had a societal shift in our attitude, we would have more understanding and support to approach and manage the process better.

So how do we change cultural perceptions of menopause in our world? We start at the grass-roots level: that means you and me. By first addressing our own perception and understanding of menopause. How is yours shaping up?

By reading this book, you've worked on understanding menopause through the management of menopausal symptoms via various treatment options, including self-care strategies. Once you've found your balance and are managing the biological, psychological and spiritual transition, it's time to look beyond the madness of perimenopause. How do you want to be perceived? How do you want these years to look? #empowered sounds like a plan to me.

These are our #wisdomyears, our time to lead our families and communities.

Humans are one of only a handful of animals that live beyond their childbearing years. Among that small but elite group are killer whales, which have an excellent reason to stop reproducing: male and female offspring stay with their mothers for life (OMG kill me now!) If she continued giving birth, the young would compete with her own direct descendants for resources such as food.[134]

So she makes the ultimate mother sacrifice by giving up her reproductive powers; no longer competing with her daughters for mating opportunities and protecting her existing offspring and grand-offspring. She carries a wealth of knowledge about where to find food, offering huge value to the pod's survival. Her genes continue on, as does her knowledge.

'One way post-reproductive females may boost the survival of their kin is through the transfer of ecological knowledge,' says Lauren Brent of the University of Exeter. 'The value gained from the wisdom of elders can help explain why female killer whales and humans continue to live long after they have stopped reproducing.'[135]

This is known as the *grandmother hypothesis*, where an older woman helps her grandchildren thrive. After menopause, she devotes her time and accumulated knowledge to help her descendants.

The anthropologist Kristen Hawkes gathered the first hard evidence of this hypothesis. Studying the Hadza people, a group of hunter-gatherers in northern Tanzania, she found that an energetic group of older women brought more food into camp than any other age and sex category.[136] So elders gained more status within the group dynamic. Fascinating stuff.

So is menopause a key to our success as a species? I think we can claim a strong argument for that. That's a great reason to embrace your renewal years and to push healthcare professionals for the treatment that's right for you. You aren't just doing it for yourself, but for humankind.

What do we want?

A change in attitude towards menopause and midlife.

When do we want it?

Now! We need advocates for change, to birth this new perception of what menopause means. This means YOU.

Let's get empowered together.

Change your language and perceptions to change the perceptions of others.

How?

Get active, vocal and creative on social media and in your communities, at your doctor's surgery, local interest groups, with your member of parliament or government at all levels, if you want to lobby for change to menopause policies in the workplace.

Talk about it with other women, daughters, sons, sisters, brothers, friends and colleagues; it doesn't have to be taboo.

By embracing our personal transition and sharing our experience, strength and hope, we become advocates for change within society. We are better placed to lobby and challenge health professionals and workplaces for more understanding and less prejudice. But we also empower our societies; women, especially the wiser older women, are surely the bedrock of all societies.

The loss of our menstrual years should offer us freedom. It's time to consider what else we can let go of, along with the tampons and period pain, to embrace the next part of our lives. Let's start believing it's a beginning and not an end, starting today.

What does this look like for you? Maybe you're one of those gracefully aged Instagram influencers, with perfectly groomed sleek grey hair bending into brilliantly flexible yoga positions, in your vintage Gucci, looking all kinds of glamorous. An aspirational grandmother type, not one wearing absorbent knickers. Or maybe you're something else entirely. You decide!

Share your menopause story with us in the **Secret Menses Business Facebook group***. I want to see all you beautiful, empowered women on social media using these hashtags #rockingmymidlife #secretmensesbusiness #wisewomenrising and standing tall and proud. Own it.

Susanne x

---

*https://www.facebook.com/groups/secretmensesbusiness

PS. If you think this book would help a friend or loved one, then please share this with them: https://www.susanne-mitchell.com/perimenopause-free-sneak-preview and I'll send them their own copy of the FREE version to get them started, direct to their inbox. Let's own it together.

Acknowledgements

While working on a book proposal for my soon-to-be-published book, *The Naked Truth About YOU*, and trying to establish my credibility as an author, I wanted to give something useful away to my readership.

A colleague in my co-work office asked me to define my readers' biggest headache. Pff! Easy. I immediately came up with a bunch of problems all related to women like me. Mid-life Generation-X, stretched between work, raising kids and caring for elderly parents, being everything to everyone else yet haunted by who we might have been as we stare 50 in the face.

He raised an eyebrow as I flicked on the kettle and continued. The reality of trying to do it all for so long has hit us hard and our discontent grows, often exacerbated the onset of health issues, reading glasses and sagging jawlines. The stress of trying to remain on the career ladder while Millennials with youthful exuberance climb over us, relationship issues and divorce, dating again, childcare for smalls and parenting teenagers only scratches the surface. How many problems do you need, Mick? I know, right?

"Susanne, you need to offer readers a headache pill that fixes an immediate problem, not a vitamin pill. What's a problem you've recently faced?"

And there it was, staring me in my just-turned-50 face. My very real and very recent battle with perimenopause and finding the answers and help I needed. I wish I had known back then what I've since discovered. So I figured I would write a short report, something that offered useful tips and information. Thank you to Mick Mooney for pushing me towards it.

Three weeks later, I was still writing and had sent it to my long-suffering and brilliant editor, Jessica Perini, who sent it back with encouraging notes to write more. As a mid-life woman, she wanted the full story. Thank you, Jess, for your friendship and ongoing mentorship, I'm a better writer because of you.

Weeks turned to months as I wrote and researched what has now become this book. Thanks to my fellow co-workers at Fourteen40, Richard Rasdall, Jennie-Lee Van Gelder and James Nosworthy for your kindness, patience and for stopping me from tearing my mid-life hair out with frustration as I encountered medical politics and delays.

Thank you to Candace Johnson, my editor in the USA, for your patience and ongoing encouragement with the proposal for my bigger book and for working out how to give part of this one away. You appeared at pivotal moments, kept pushing me in all the right directions, and I'm so grateful to call you my friend. To Caroline Webber for taking over from Jess at short notice and providing much-needed publishing savvy and direction, thank you. And to Zena Shapter, who saved the day and my sanity through the e-book production, more edits and an eleventh-hour decision to create a print version. To Anita Henderson, who provided my website, offering much patience and help with setting up mailing list processes and endless design headaches.

It's strange how almost everyone who helped and supported me were mid-life women in varying stages of peri- or postmenopause with experiences to share. Your support and belief in the project has been so important to me. There were more; thank you to Valerie McIver, my

PR guru, for a cool head, calm influence and friendship, and to Sam McFarlane and Amy Wyhoon for social smarts and patience with my extended deadlines.

Thank you to Reza Bagheri for kindly fixing my mis-matched PR photos at short notice, without removing my wrinkles or grey roots, tempting though it was. And to Peter Morley for your professional book cover design skills and answering my endless questions about colour profiles.

Recognising Arts Law for the important work it does in Australia on behalf of artists and creative communities, we are very fortunate to have this organisation and its volunteers. Vincent Floro, you kindly offered me expert pro-bono advice as part of Arts Law's Document Review Service, I'm so very grateful for your time and help.

I was lucky to talk directly with so many medical professionals through my personal experience and research, thank you to Dr. Tim Tregonning and Dr. Kate Ilbery for your ongoing help and support, Michael Buckley, Associate Professor John Eden, Professor Susan Davis and Dr. Darshika Christie-David. Thank you Miia Prowse for your naturopathic expertise and kindness. And to all those whose medical research I laboured through to understand as a non-medical person, your work is vital, thank you. To Dr. Rebecca Glaser and Dr. Angela DeRosa, I am so grateful for your knowledge and insight, you were both what the doctor ordered at a point where I had given up looking for the other side to the story.

I'm also grateful to my ex-husband Danny Mitchell for stepping in to help when life bit my perimenopausal-arse at times, and for your loving parenting of our kids. To Becca Mitchell for finding time to read my work. Thanks to my sister Jaki, her husband Pete, Mum and Dad, Harry, Sonia, Bethany, James, Rosie and Rhys for being there through this awful year, to show me how important my family are to me, via

Zoom and WhatsApp from the UK. I love waking up to a gazillion messages about what you all ate yesterday or grew in the veggie patch. Miss you.

To Darren Bender, your ongoing love and friendship is gold, thank you. And for all my girlfriends, new ones like Lynda Babister, Alison Sutton, Claire Steinke, Victoria Fox, Simone Spender, Jan Taylor, Lyn Storey, Margie Connelly and longtime-friends, Phillippa Andrew, Rita Mann, Nikki Cronin, Robyn Plunkett, Jane Ewen and Claire Killick, we've been through many adventures together, your love, laughs and ongoing support mean the world to me. Bless.

To Nick Mansell for holding me steady in your heart, for setting a course for us both through such tumultuous seas, and for believing in me when I couldn't manage it for myself. I'm excited to become your wife, thank you for asking me. Slow-blink. Finally, to Ella and Rowan, you constantly inspire me to be a better human and to keep aiming for infinity and beyond. I don't know how I got so lucky to be your Mama. I love you.

About the Author

Susanne Mitchell is a writer, media professional and self-professed kitchen sink philosopher. She has helped businesses share authentic stories through written and video content via her own small media consultancy.

Susanne has 30 years of experience working with broadcasters, including the BBC, Disney, ABC Australia and NBC America on feature films, documentaries and television drama. Though she turned down the opportunity to work with Sir David Attenborough at the BBC's Natural History Unit – a youthful decision she laments – Susanne has mingled with movie stars and travelled with the legendary former Australian prime minister Bob Hawke.

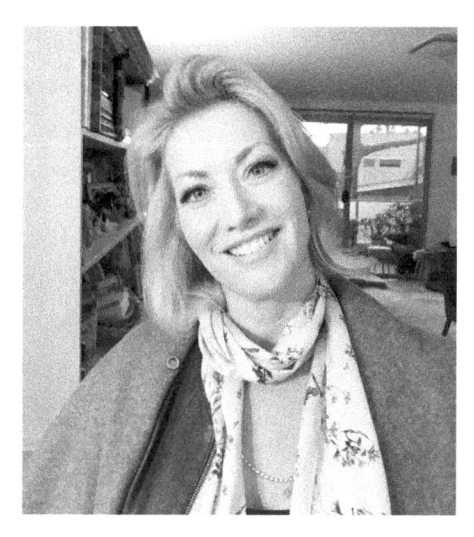

Photo: Ella Mitchell

Daughter-in-law to the late Warren Mitchell, a British actor best known for playing Alf Garnet in *Til Death do Us Part*, she admits he played an important role through her 20s and 30s. Encouraging Susanne to expand her understanding of the world, Warren challenged her to have the courage of her convictions and to seek the truth, a pursuit that heavily influences her work.

A creative storyteller who now calls Australia home, Susanne is interested in the human condition and will engage with anyone and everyone in her search for answers to our greatest challenge – how to live a life of purpose while contributing to society and reaching our highest potential.

Her second book, *The Naked Truth About YOU, Unlock the secret to a kick-arse life*, will be released in late 2021. It's a refreshing and compelling look at today's hottest self-development topics that weaves a potent thread of philosophy, psychology, and neuroscience through an engaging narrative of true stories.

Using her own life experiences and living with type 1 diabetes, Susanne is an ordinary, insulin pump-wearing woman on a quest to improve who we are and how we choose to live. This mother of two young adults currently resides in Sydney with her partner Nick, son Rowan, two Burmese cat-dogs and a rescue hound called Crumpet.

The Naked Truth About YOU

Unlock the secret to a kick-arse life
Also by Susanne Mitchell

The Naked Truth About YOU is one woman's search for answers to our greatest challenge: how to create a life of purpose, love, connection while contributing to society and reaching your highest potential.

But living in our over-scheduled world, managing family, careers, technology, and ongoing stress, many people find there's simply nothing left to give. How can we possibly achieve a worthwhile life?

In this refreshing and compelling look at today's hottest self-development topics, Susanne Mitchell – writer, storyteller, kitchen sink philosopher and media professional – weaves a potent thread of philosophy, psychology, and neuroscience through an engaging narrative of true stories.

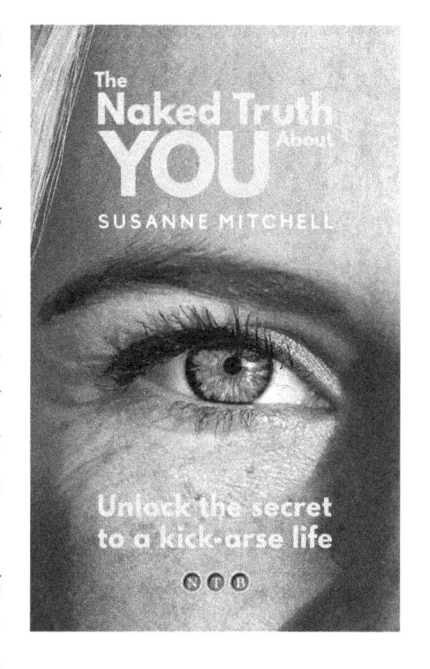

Using humour, profound insight, and an easygoing down-to-earth wisdom, Susanne reveals her innermost secrets while encouraging you to disrobe and take an honest look at your own naked truth.

The knowledge she shares in *The Naked Truth About YOU* will guide you to understand what fuels your everyday actions, thoughts and emotions. She demonstrates how increased self-awareness offers the freedom to live a truly authentic life.

After hitting her middle years weighed down by the overwhelming demands of life, depression, divorce and chronic disease, Susanne took a dramatic face-plant into crisis.

Her choices were to give up the fight and live in beige-toned mediocrity while quietly falling apart, or shed her heavy superwoman cape to understand who she really was underneath the bluff and bravado.

What are the vital and elusive ingredients to creating a kick-arse life? Courageously pulling on her big-girl knickers, Susanne shares the secrets she discovered with you.

*

It's brilliant. Gripping. Insight filled. Moving. Funny. Empathetic. Heart breaking. Hair-raising. Entertaining and surprisingly funny. Reading this book is a big experience. It's a profound take on the most important subject facing humans now. Having something clear, fresh, relevant, and powerful to say about it is not a small thing. This book is very important. It might save lives. No, it will save lives. And it will change lives.

Darren Bender

Lone Wolf Pictures, TV producer and former commissioning editor Channel 4 Television

*

'If I had read the book a few years ago I think I could have sorted a few things and enjoyed the last few years instead of suffering crippling self-doubt, with the inevitable inertia that comes from not getting another perspective on what is happening and why it is happening to me.'

*

'I've finished your book and I loved it, what a beautifully crafted piece of work. Your storytelling is so visual, and that's a really enjoyable way to read.'

*

'You've made me laugh, cry and think. And that thinking has undoubtedly brought up a lot of great perspective and things to utilise in my life.'
#stopworrying #bemorelikepooh #acceptance

*

'Your story in particular is compelling and I think many, many people can relate to the inner struggles and how they manifest to external struggles until we work through them.'

www.susanne-mitchell.com

If you'd like to receive a FREE preview chapter, please head to www.susanne-mitchell.com/the-naked-truth-about-you-preview/

https://www.facebook.com/susannemitchellauthor/

https://www.instagram.com/kitchensinkphilosopher/

https://www.facebook.com/groups/secretmensesbusiness

Resources

Rock My Menopause is the public-face of the UK's Primary Care Women's Health Forum (PCWHF), a group of 10,000 healthcare professionals with a special interest in women's health. It has some great fact sheets and information: https://rockmymenopause.com/

Don't forget that medical societies are potentially conflicted by their affiliations, but they are also a very useful resource with lots of useful information. Use them.

International Menopause Society
https://www.imsociety.org/

Australasian Menopause Society
www.menopause.org.au

European Menopause and Andropause Society (EMAS)
www.emas-online.org

The German Menopause Society
www.menopause-gesellschaft.de

The Jean Hailes Foundation

www.jeanhailes.org.au

National Women's Health Resource Center

www.healthywomen.org

North American Menopause Society

www.menopause.org

University of Melbourne Key Centre for Women's Health in Society

www.kcwh.unimelb.edu.au

The Women's Health Council (Ireland)

www.nwci.ie

Menopause Matters

www.menopausematters.co.uk

The Global Library of Women's Medicine

www.glowm.com

The British Menopause Society

www.thebms.org.uk

Definitions of Menopause Terminology are clearly stated by the IMS here: https://www.imsociety.org/menopause_terminology.php.

Perimenopause

https://www.menopause.org.au/hp/information-sheets/1057-perimenopause

https://www.jeanhailes.org.au/resources/perimenopause-fact-sheet

https://www.health.harvard.edu/womens-health/perimenopause-rocky-road-to-menopause

HRT/MHT

https://www.womens-health-concern.org/wp-content/uploads/2020/03/WHC-FACTSHEET-HRT-BenefitsRisks-MAR2020.pdf

https://rockmymenopause.com/wp-content/uploads/2019/06/HRT-Myths-Uncovered.pdf

https://www.menopause.org.au/images/factsheets/What_is_MHT_and_is_it_safe_V7.pdf

Testosterone

www.menopause.org.au/health-info/resources/1484-testosterone-and-women

www.menopause.org.au/images/docs/Testosterone_and_Women.pdf

https://www.womens-health-concern.org/help-and-advice/factsheets/testosterone-for-women/

www.menopause.org.au/hp/position-statements/1469-international-consensus-on-testosterone-treatment-for-women

A Woman's Hormonal Health Survival Guide: How to Prevent Your Doctor from Slowly Killing You by Dr. Angela DeRosa, DO MBA CPE. Highly recommended reading.

Endnotes

1 https://rockmymenopause.com/get-informed/menopause/ Rock My Menopause is a campaign of the Primary Care Women's Health Forum (PCWHF) in the UK, a group of 10,000 healthcare professionals with a special interest in women's health. [accessed 26 May 2020]

2 https://www.monash.edu/__data/assets/pdf_file/0005/1003397/testosterone-patient-information-sheet.pdf [accessed 21 August 2020]

3 https://www.menopause.org.au/hp/information-sheets/1057-perimenopause [accessed 25 August 2020]

4 https://www.womens-health-concern.org/help-and-advice/factsheets/menopause/ [accessed 21 August 2020]

5 https://www.imsociety.org/manage/images/pdf/a0342d018487cfc9744445c5af7c49ad.pdf fact sheet states: 'On average, perimenopause will last four years.' However this academic paper states 1–3 years: https://www.ncbi.nlm.nih.gov/pmc/articles/PMC3580996/ 'LATE MENOPAUSAL TRANSITION (Stage −1) Based on studies of menstrual calendars and on changes in FSH and estradiol, this stage is estimated to last on average 1-3 years. Symptoms, most notably vasomotor symptoms, are likely to occur during this stage.' [accessed 21 August 2020]

6   https://rockmymenopause.com/get-informed/menopause/ Dr Jane Davis: 'Did you know? Symptoms can start a good 10 years before your last period. If you think your hormones are changing then they are probably changing. Remember, you know your own body best.' [accessed 21 August 2020]

7   https://www.womens-health-concern.org/help-and-advice/factsheets/menopause/ [accessed 21 August 2020]

8   Personal correspondence with Dr. Angela DeRosa, October 2020.

9   https://www.monash.edu/news/articles/menopause-symptoms-are-associated-with-poor-self-assessed-work-ability [accessed 21 August 2020] 'Common symptoms of menopause include: hot flushes and night sweats, disrupted sleep; anxiety and disturbed mood; and joint pain.' https://www.menopause.org.au/health-info/fact-sheets/menopause-what-are-the-symptoms [accessed 21 August 2020] https://rockmymenopause.com/wp-content/uploads/2019/05/RMM_Symptoms.pdf [accessed 21 August 2020] Professor Susan Davis advised me in August 2020 that weight gain is not a common symptom of menopause but central abdominal fat gain is. Weight gain is attributed to aging. Personally I gained weight EVERYWHERE through perimenopause.

10 https://rockmymenopause.com/get-informed/menopause/ [accessed 26 May 2020]

11 https://www.monash.edu/medicine/sphpm/units/womenshealth/info-4-health-practitioners/testosterone-for-women [accessed 21 August 2020]

12 https://www.ncbi.nlm.nih.gov/books/NBK279388/ [accessed 28 September 2020]

13 DeRosa, Angela. How Your Doctor is Slowly Killing You. DeRosa Media. Chapter One e-book 2018

14 Personal correspondence with Dr. Angela DeRosa, October 2020.

15 https://www.hormone.org/your-health-and-hormones/glands-and-hormones-a-to-z/hormones/estrogen [accessed 26 August 2020]

16 https://www.hormone.org/your-health-and-hormones/glands-and-hormones-a-to-z/hormones/estrone

17 https://lens.monash.edu/@medicine-health/2019/11/18/1378410/making-sense-of-menopausal-hormone-therapy-means-understanding-the-benefits-as-well-as-the-risks-susan-davis-chair-of-womens-health-monash-university [accessed 26 August 2020]

18 https://www.health.harvard.edu/womens-health/dealing-with-the-symptoms-of-menopause [accessed 31 July 2020]

19 DeRosa, Angela. How Your Doctor is Slowly Killing You. DeRosa Media. Chapter One e-book 2018

20 Personal correspondence with Dr. Angela DeRosa, October 2020.

21 https://lens.monash.edu/@medicine-health/2019/11/18/1378410/making-sense-of-menopausal-hormone-therapy-means-understanding-the-benefits-as-well-as-the-risks-susan-davis-chair-of-womens-health-monash-university [accessed 26 August 2020]

22 https://www.ncbi.nlm.nih.gov/pmc/articles/PMC5327627/ Szamatowicz M. How can gynaecologists cope with the silent killer – osteoporosis? Prz Menopauzalny. 2016; 15(4): 189–192. doi:10.5114/pm.2016.65682 [accessed 26 August 2020]

23 https://www.hormone.org/your-health-and-hormones/glands-and-hormones-a-to-z/hormones/progesterone [accessed 31 July 2020]

24 https://www.menopause.org.au/images/docs/Changes_before_the_Change.pdf [accessed 31 July 2020]

25 https://lens.monash.edu/@medicine-health/2019/11/18/1378410/making-sense-of-menopausal-hormone-therapy-means-understanding-the-benefits-as-well-as-the-risks-susan-davis-chair-of-womens-health-monash-university [accessed 26 August 2020]

26 https://www.hormone.org/your-health-and-hormones/glands-and-hormones-a-to-z/hormones/progesterone [accessed 21 August 2020]

27 Professor Eden prescribes me a combined product of bioidentical hormones, Estradiol and Prometrium. They cost around $50 a pack of both hormones (in Australia) rather than around $40 each as separate items. It's called Estrogel Pro Combination pack.

28 Personal correspondence with Dr. Angela DeRosa, October 2020.

29 https://www.monash.edu/__data/assets/pdf_file/0005/1003397/testosterone-patient-information-sheet.pdf [accessed 21 August 2020]

30 Dr. Rebecca Glaser, presentation Saturday 12th September 2020 via Zoom Androgen Decline and Aging Presentation (Powerpoint) recording available here: https://www.trocarkit.com/pages/presentations accessed 2 October 2020

31 Personal correspondence with Dr. Angela DeRosa, October 2020.

32 Personal correspondence with Dr. Angela DeRosa, October 2020.

33 https://www.maturitas.org/article/S0378-5122(13)00012-1/pdf [accessed 26 August 2020] Glaser, Rebecca and Dimitrakakis, Constantine (2013) Testosterone therapy in women: Myths and misconceptions Maturitas https://doi.org/10.1016/j.maturitas.2013.01.003

34 DeRosa, Angela, DO MBA CPE. How Your Doctor is Slowly Killing You: A Woman's Hormonal Health Survival Guide. DeRosa Media 2018.

35 This is the author's personal experience and there are many differences of opinion in the medical world over testosterone having any effect on cognitive function or fatigue.

36 https://www.ncbi.nlm.nih.gov/books/NBK279388/ [accessed 28 September 2020]

37 DeRosa, Angela, DO MBA CPE. How Your Doctor is Slowly Killing You: A Woman's Hormonal Health Survival Guide. DeRosa Media 2018.

38 Wilson RA. Feminine Forever – the amazing new breakthrough in the sex life of women. New York: Evans, 1966.

39 https://pubmed.ncbi.nlm.nih.gov/12649555/ [accessed 26 August 2020] Houck JA. 'What do these women want?': Feminist responses to Feminine Forever, 1963–1980. Bull Hist Med. 2003; 77(1): 103–132. doi:10.1353/bhm.2003.0023

40 https://www.latimes.com/archives/la-xpm-1994-08-09-ls-25315-story.html [accessed 26 August 2020]

41 https://www.ncbi.nlm.nih.gov/pmc/articles/PMC6780820 [accessed 26 August 2020]

42 https://pubmed.ncbi.nlm.nih.gov/12649555/ [accessed 26 August 2020] Houck JA. 'What do these women want?': Feminist responses to Feminine Forever, 1963–1980. Bull Hist Med. 2003; 77(1): 103–132. doi:10.1353/bhm.2003.0023

43 Manderson et al, 'Circuit Breaking: Pathways of Treatment Seeking for Women with Endometriosis in Australia', Qualitative Health Research 18:4 (2008), page 532 https://www.theguardian.com/lifeandstyle/2019/nov/13/the-female-problem-male-bias-in-medical-trials [accessed 20 October 2020]

44 https://www.bhf.org.uk/what-we-do/news-from-the-bhf/news-archive/2018/november/8000-uk-women-die-due-to-unequal-heart-attack-care [accessed 20 October 2020]

45 DeRosa, Angela, DO MBA CPE. How Your Doctor is Slowly Killing You: A Woman's Hormonal Health Survival Guide. DeRosa Media 2018. Location 433.

46 https://www.ncbi.nlm.nih.gov/pmc/articles/PMC5415400/ [accessed 31 July 2020] Vogel L. Trial overstated HRT risk for younger women. CMAJ. 2017; 189(17): E648–E649. doi:10.1503/cmaj.1095421

47 https://www.ncbi.nlm.nih.gov/pmc/articles/PMC5415400/ [accessed 31 July 2020]

48 https://www.womens-health-concern.org/help-and-advice/factsheets/hrt-know-benefits-risks/ [accessed 31 July 2020] In July 2012 Women's Health Concern formally became the patient arm of British Menopause Society (BMS)

49 https://www.ncbi.nlm.nih.gov/pmc/articles/PMC5415400/ [accessed 31 July 2020]

50 https://www.ncbi.nlm.nih.gov/pmc/articles/PMC5415400/ [accessed 31 July 2020]

51 https://www.tandfonline.com/doi/abs/10.1080/13697130310001651418 [accessed 31 July 2020] Samuel Shapiro (2004) The Million Women Study: potential biases do not allow uncritical acceptance of the data, Climacteric, 7:1, 3-7, DOI: 10.1080/13697130310001651418

52 https://thebms.org.uk/2017/03/new-paper-professor-robert-d-langer-demonstrates-whi-study-errors-led-15-years-unnecessary-suffering-women/ [accessed 31 July 2020]

53 Sarah Boseley, 'HRT won't kill you – but menopausal women still face a difficult decision', 16 September 2017, https://www.theguardian.com/society/2017/sep/15/hrt-hormone-replacement-therapy-wont-kill-you-but-menopausal-women-still-face-a-difficult-decision and https://jamanetwork.com/journals/jama/fullarticle/2653735 [accessed 31 July 2020]

54 https://www.womens-health-concern.org/help-and-advice/factsheets/hrt-know-benefits-risks/ [accessed 31 July 2020]

55 NICE Guidelines [NG23] 2015 https://rockmymenopause.com/wp-content/uploads/2019/06/HRT-Myths-Uncovered.pdf [accessed 31 July 2020]

56 www.womens-health-concern.org/wp-content/uploads/2020/03/WHC-FACTSHEET-HRT-BenefitsRisks-MAR2020.pdf [accessed 31 July 2020]

57 www.ncbi.nlm.nih.gov/pmc/articles/PMC5415400/ [accessed 31 July 2020]

58 https://pubmed.ncbi.nlm.nih.gov/23865654/ [accessed 31 July 2020] Sarrel PM, Njike VY, Vinante V, Katz DL. The mortality toll of estrogen avoidance: an analysis of excess deaths among hysterectomized women aged 50 to 59 years. Am J Public Health. 2013; 103(9): 1583–1588. doi:10.2105/AJPH.2013.301295

59 https://www1.racgp.org.au/newsgp/clinical/what-should-gps-know-about-compounded-bioidentical [accessed 28 August 2020]

60 https://core.ac.uk/download/pdf/187931831.pdf [accessed 21 October 2021]

61 https://www1.racgp.org.au/newsgp/clinical/what-should-gps-know-about-compounded-bioidentical [accessed 28 September 2020]

62 DeRosa, Angela stated this in an interview via Zoom 29 September 2020

63 https://www.whria.com.au/co2-fractional-laser-treatment-for-vaginal-atrophy-4/ [accessed 7 October 2020]

64 https://www1.racgp.org.au/newsgp/clinical/what-should-gps-know-about-compounded-bioidentical [accessed 28 August 2020]

65 DeRosa, Angela, DO MBA CPE. How Your Doctor is Slowly Killing You: A Woman's Hormonal Health Survival Guide. E-book location 575 DeRosa Media 2018.

66 https://www.pharmacyregulation.org/standards/standards-registered-pharmacies [accessed 21 October 2020]

67 Personal correspondence with Dr. Angela DeRosa, October 2020.

68 https://www1.racgp.org.au/newsgp/clinical/what-should-gps-know-about-compounded-bioidentical [accessed 28 August 2020]

69 DeRosa, Angela, DO MBA CPE. How Your Doctor is Slowly Killing You: A Woman's Hormonal Health Survival Guide. E-book location 506. DeRosa Media 2018.

70 DeRosa, Angela, DO MBA CPE. How Your Doctor is Slowly Killing You: A Woman's Hormonal Health Survival Guide. DeRosa Media 2018.

71 www.medicines.org.uk/emc/product/1597/pil [accessed 31 July 2020] 'Your body breaks down tibolone to make hormones'

72 www.menopause.org.au/images/stories/infosheets/docs/AMS_Tibolone_for_post-menopausal_women_April_2015.pdf [accessed 31 July 2020]

73 https://www.menopause.org.au/hp/information-sheets/1287-tibolone-as-menopausal-hormone-therapy [accessed 31 July 2020] references this paper; https://pubmed.ncbi.nlm.nih.gov/19167925/ [accessed 31 July

2020] Kenemans P, Bundred NJ, Foidart JM, Kubista E, von Schoultz B, Sismondi P, et al. LIBERATE Study Group. Safety and efficacy of tibolone in breast-cancer patients with vasomotor symptoms: a double-blind, randomised, noninferiority trial. Lancet Oncology 2009; 10(2): 135–146

74 www.menopause.org.au/hp/information-sheets/1287-tibolone-as-menopausal-hormone-therapy [accessed 31 July 2020]

75 www.menopause.org.au/images/stories/infosheets/docs/AMS_Tibolone_for_post-menopausal_women_April_2015.pdf [accessed 31 July 2020]

76 http://www.imperial.ac.uk/news/185248/new-class-menopause-drugs-reduces-severity [accessed 31 July 2020] Professor Waljit Dhillo study author: 'This class of new drugs may provide women with a much-needed alternative to HRT'

77 https://www.mja.com.au/journal/2002/176/3/ethical-issues-concerning-relationships-between-medical-practitioners-and [accessed 3 October 2020]

78 https://www.chronicle.com/article/the-secret-lives-of-big-pharmas-thought-leaders/ [accessed 3 October 2020]

79 https://www.chronicle.com/article/the-secret-lives-of-big-pharmas-thought-leaders/ [accessed 3 October 2020]

80 Sismondo, Sergio, 'You're Not Just a Paid Monkey Reading Slides:' How Key Opinion Leaders Explain and Justify Their Work (October 10, 2013). Edmond J. Safra Working Papers, No. 26, Available at SSRN: https://ssrn.com/abstract=2338704 [accessed 3 October 2020]

81 https://www.imsociety.org/ethical_codes_of_conduct.php [accessed 3 October 2020]

82 BMJ 2015;350:h2942 doi: 10.1136/bmj.h2942 (Published 2 June 2015) https://www.bmj.com/content/350/bmj.h2942 [accessed 3 October 2020]

83 This will vary between individual women. www.monash.edu/medicine/sphpm/units/womenshealth/info-4-health-practitioners/testosterone-for-women [accessed 31 July 2020]

84 In conversation with Dr. Angela DeRosa, 30th September 2020 via Zoom.

85 https://www.menopause.org/docs/default-document-library/hsddkingsberg.pdf?sfvrsn=2 [accessed 28 August 2020]

86 https://www.sciencedirect.com/science/article/pii/S0378512213000121#! [accessed 31 July 2020] Testosterone therapy in women: Myths and misconceptions, Glaser R. Dimitrakakis C. (2013) Maturitas, 74 (3), 230–234.

87 https://www.womens-health-concern.org/help-and-advice/factsheets/testosterone-for-women/ [accessed 7 September 2020] Blood tests are not able to diagnose whether or not you need testosterone but are used as a safety check to ensure you are not getting too much on top of your own natural levels; http://www.menopause.org.au/images/docs/Testosterone_and_Women.pdf [accessed 31 July 2020] The effects of low testosterone in women have been greatly debated over many years. Firstly, and most importantly there is no blood level that can be used as a cut-off to "diagnose" low testosterone in women.

88 https://www.sciencedirect.com/science/article/pii/S0378512213000121#! [accessed 31 July 2020] Testosterone therapy in women: Myths and misconceptions, Glaser R. Dimitrakakis C. (2013) Maturitas, 74 (3), 230–234. [accessed 2nd October 2020] 'Safety, tolerability and clinical response should guide therapy rather than a single T measurement, which is extremely variable and inherently unreliable.'

89 https://www.sciencedirect.com/science/article/pii/S0378512213000121#! [accessed 31 July 2020] Testosterone therapy in women: Myths and misconceptions, Glaser R. Dimitrakakis C. (2013) Maturitas, 74 (3), 230–234. [accessed 2nd October 2020] and R. Glaser, A. York & C.

Dimitrakakis (2016) Effect of testosterone therapy on the female voice, Climacteric, 19:2, 198-203, DOI: 10.3109/13697137.2015.1136925

90 https://www.womens-health-concern.org/wp-content/uploads/2020/04/WHC-FACTSHEET-Testosterone-for-women-APR2020.pdf [accessed 31 July 2020]

91 https://www.menopause.org.au/images/docs/ICMT_A_1637079_O.pdf and https://docs.google.com/document/d/10TyA8o9uFSs-8ZFvl7zulISTtLi0jifQll5ElLw_Mhg/edit [accessed 31 July 2020]

92 Ross JS. Randomized Clinical Trials and Observational Studies Are More Often Alike Than Unlike. JAMA Intern Med. 2014;174(10):1557. doi:10.1001/jamainternmed.2014.3366

93 Anglemyer A, Horvath HT, Bero L. Healthcare outcomes assessed with observational study designs compared with those assessed in randomized trials. Cochrane Database Syst Rev. 2014;4:MR000034.

94 https://academic.oup.com/jcem/article-abstract/105/6/e2308/5803242 [accessed 3 October 2020] Letter to the Editor: "Global Consensus Position Statement on the Use of Testosterone Therapy for Women" A Edward Friedman The Journal of Clinical Endocrinology & Metabolism, Volume 105, Issue 6, June 2020, pages e2308 e2309, https://doi.org/10.1210/clinem/dgaa118 and in personal communication with Dr. Rebecca Glaser M.D. FACS September 2020.

95 In personal communication with Dr. Rebecca Glaser M.D. FACS September 2020.

96 https://www.thelancet.com/journals/landia/article/PIIS2213-8587(19)30189-5 [accessed 31 July 2020] Islam RM, Bell RJ, Green S, Page MJ, Davis, SR. Safety and efficacy of testosterone for women: a systematic review and meta-analysis of randomised controlled trial data. The Lancet Diabetes & Endocrinology. 25 July 2019.

97 Glaser, Rebecca et al. Beneficial effects of testosterone therapy in women measured by the validated Menopause Rating Scale (MRS) Maturitas, Volume 68, Issue 4, 355 - 361

98 www.monash.edu/medicine/news/latest/2019-articles/large-study-shows-beneficial-role-of-testosterone-for-postmenopausal-women [accessed 31 July 2020]

99 In personal communication with Michael Buckley, MD of Lawley Pharmaceuticals in WA, Australia on 26 November 2020. The quote by Professor Davis is clearly stated in the Lawley Press Release dated 20 November 2020 sent to me via email by Mr. Buckley. You can read more from that release reported here: https://www.menopausedoctor.co.uk/news/testosterone-now-licensed-for-women-in-australia [accessed 30 November 2020]

100 www.menopause.org.au/hp/information-sheets/600-nonhormonal-treatments-for-menopausal-symptoms [accessed 31 July 2020]

101 https://www.beyondblue.org.au/get-support/get-immediate-support [accessed 28 August 2020] We all have good days and bad days. Then there are those days when something isn't quite right, you've got something on your mind, or things just seem too much. Whatever it may be, sharing the load with someone else can really help. If you need to talk things through with someone start here (in Australia) or search Google for a helpline in your country.

102 www.menopause.org.au/health-info/fact-sheets/non-hormonal-treatment-options-for-menopausal-symptoms [accessed 31 July 2020]

103 Rada G, Capurro D, Pantoja T, Corbalán J, Moreno G, Letelier LM, Vera C. Non-hormonal interventions for hot flushes in women with a history of breast cancer. Cochrane Database of Systematic Reviews 2010, Issue 9. Art. No: CD004923. DOI: 10.1002/14651858.CD004923.pub2.

104 https://www.menopause.org.au/health-info/fact-sheets/non-hormonal-treatment-options-for-menopausal-symptoms [accessed 31 July 2020]

105 https://www.ncbi.nlm.nih.gov/pmc/articles/PMC5611767/ [accessed 28 August 2020] Melatonin in perimenopausal and postmenopausal women: associations with mood, sleep, climacteric symptoms, and quality of life. Toffol E, Kalleinen N, Haukka J, Vakkuri O, Partonen T, Polo-Kantola P. Menopause. 2014 May; 21(5): 493–500.

106 https://www.sciencedaily.com/releases/2018/09/180905083901.htm [accessed 31 July 2020]

107 Betz JM, Anderson L, Avigan MI, Barnes J, Farnsworth NR, Gerdén B, et al. Black cohosh: considerations of safety and benefit. Nutr Today 2009; 44: 155–162.

108 Foster S. Black cohosh: a literature review. HerbalGram 1999; 45: 35–50.

109 www.cochranelibrary.com/cdsr/doi/10.1002/14651858.CD007244.pub2/full?highlightAbstract=cohosh%7Cblack [accessed 31 July 2020]. Cochrane Review found adequate justification for conducting further studies on black cohosh's use to treat menopausal symptoms due to the uncertain quality of most studies included in the review.

110 https://ods.od.nih.gov/factsheets/BlackCohosh-HealthProfessional/ 'Warning: Black cohosh may harm the liver in some individuals. Use under the supervision of a healthcare professional' [accessed 31 July 2020]

111 www.menopause.org.au/images/stories/infosheets/docs/AMS_Complementary_and_Herbal_Medicines_Hot_Flushes.pdf [accessed 31 July 2020]

112 www.menopause.org.au/images/stories/infosheets/docs/AMS_Complementary_and_Herbal_Medicines_Hot_Flushes.pdf [accessed 31 July 2020]

113 www.menopause.org.au/images/stories/infosheets/docs/AMS_Complementary_and_Herbal_Medicines_Hot_Flushes.pdf [accessed 31 July 2020]

114 Maca-JDS was patented in 2018 and doesn't appear to be available in any commercial products; www.cochranelibrary.com/central/doi/10.1002/central/CN-01784659/full#information [accessed 1 September 2020]

115 www.menopause.org.au/images/stories/infosheets/docs/AMS_Complementary_and_Herbal_Medicines_Hot_Flushes.pdf [accessed 31 July 2020]

116 https://www.cochranelibrary.com/central/doi/10.1002/central/CN-02077984/full [accessed 1 September 2020]

117 https://www.menopause.org.au/images/stories/infosheets/docs/AMS_Complementary_and_Herbal_Medicines_Hot_Flushes.pdf [accessed 31 July 2020]

118 www.menopause.org.au/images/stories/infosheets/docs/AMS_Complementary_and_Herbal_Medicines_Hot_Flushes.pdf [accessed 31 July 2020]

119 www.menopause.org.au/images/stories/infosheets/docs/AMS_Complementary_and_Herbal_Medicines_Hot_Flushes.pdf [accessed 31 July 2020]

120 www.menopause.org.au/health-info/fact-sheets/lifestyle-and-behaviour-changes-for-menopausal-symptoms [accessed 31 July 2020]

121 Consultation with Miia Prowse BSc Adv Dip Nat MATMS, 22 June 2020.

122 This article contains useful insights on managing stress, getting good sleep, nutrition and exercise https://pathtowellness.ca/naturopathic-approach-to-managing-menopause/ Camille Nghiem-Phu, BSc, ND, 2008 [accessed 31 July 2020]

123 https://rockmymenopause.com/pelvic-floor-face [accessed 31 July 2020]

124 www.healthline.com/health/ten-best-menopause-activities#yoga-and-meditation [accessed 31 July 2020]

125 The CDC recommends that beginners start with 10 minutes of light activity, slowly boosting exercise intensity as it becomes easier. https://www.cdc.gov/physicalactivity/basics/adults/index.htm [accessed 31 July 2020]

126 https://www.ncbi.nlm.nih.gov/pmc/articles/PMC4609431/ [accessed 31 July 2020]

127 www.menopause.org.au/health-info/fact-sheets/lifestyle-and-behaviour-changes-for-menopausal-symptoms [accessed 31 July 2020]

128 International Association for Cognitive Psychotherapy – Therapist Referrals

129 Sood R, Kuhle CL, Kapoor E, et al. Association of mindfulness and stress with menopausal symptoms in midlife women. Climacteric. 2019; 22(4): 377–382. doi:10.1080/13697137.2018.1551344

130 No scientific proof exists to support adrenal fatigue as a true medical condition. However starting an exercise program, eating healthy foods, and following a daily routine for sleeping and waking will almost always make you feel better, no matter what the medical diagnosis. https://www.hormone.org/diseases-and-conditions/adrenal-fatigue [accessed 28 August 2020]

131 https://www.menopause.org/for-women/menopauseflashes/menopause-symptoms-and-treatments/how-do-i-know-i'm-in-menopause- [accessed 7 September 2020]

132 www.imsociety.org/links.php [accessed 31 July 2020]

133 E. Stefanopoulou, P. Gupta, R. Mohamed Mostafa, N. Nosair, Z. Mirghani, K. Moustafa, G. Al Kusayer, D. W. Sturdee & M. S. Hunter (2014) IMS study of Climate, Altitude, Temperature and vasomotor symptoms in the United Arab Emirates, Climacteric, 17:4, 425-432, DOI: 10.3109/13697137.2014.898266

134 https://phys.org/news/2018-08-beluga-whales-narwhals-menopause.html#jCp [accessed 31 July 2020] Samuel Ellis et al, Analyses of ovarian activity reveal repeated evolution of post-reproductive lifespans in toothed whales, Scientific Reports (2018). DOI: 10.1038/s41598-018-31047-8

135 www.smithsonianmag.com/science-nature/after-menopause-killer-whale-moms-become-pod-leaders-180954480 [accessed 31 July 2020]

136 www.npr.org/sections/goatsandsoda/2019/02/07/692088371/living-near-your-grandmother-has-evolutionary-benefits [accessed 31 July 2020]